KETO COUNTER

Where Carb Counts Come First!

A Quick Reference Guide of Keto Nutrition Facts

By

Ann Scritsmier

Table of Contents

	Page
Introduction	3-8
Vegetables	11-14
Eggs, Milk, Cream	14
Yogurt & Cheese	15
Oils, Butter, Dressings & Spreads	16
Meat & Poultry	17
Fish & Shell Food	17-18
Processed Meats	19
Legumes, Nuts & Seeds	19-20
Fruits & Fruit Juices	20-22
Breads & Grains	22-23
Sauces, Dips & Sides	23-24
Baking Ingredients & Sweeteners	24-25
Spices & Seasonings	26
Crackers & Chips	26
Desserts & Other Baked Goods	27
Beverages	27-28
Supplements	28
Foods in Alphabetical Order	31-47
Keto Friendly Recipes	51-72
Index	75-90

INTRO

About this book and what to expect....

The contents of the Keto Counter book is primarily nutritional information. This book is intended for those currently following or wanting to start a low-carb or Keto diet, although anyone can benefit from the nutritional facts in the book.

It's not intended to be a **complete** book on all foods and their nutritional info, but rather some of the more common foods you'll encounter while at home cooking, at office functions, or attending a party.

Within the nutritional facts, you will notice some high carb food items such as beans, breads, fruit juices, and desserts. Though not conducive to a ketogenic diet, they were included only to bring awareness of the carb counts in these common foods.

Food items are listed categorically and alphabetically, along with a smidgen of Keto recipes to help you get started. Under each recipe title is the website address, where the recipe can be found online for additional images or instructions.

Whenever you see a food item listed as 'single', it means literally one. For example -- 1 chip, 1 cracker, 1 nut, 1 berry, 1 apple, etc., to help you determine how many you can have of that item and keep your carb counts under control for the day.

Where vegetables are concerned, boiled counts will be similar to steamed.

I am not in the medical or health profession. I do, however, have working knowledge of the ketogenic diet, along with years of experience following a low carb diet and am a researcher at heart.

If you need medical or nutritional advice, please consult with your doctor or a certified nutritionist. A nutritionist who specializes in the ketogenic diet would be ideal. You can find many of them online.

Two of my favorite practitioners who are passionate about low carb dieting to attain and maintain good health are, **Dr. Mercola, DO** (www.mercola.com), and **Dr. Berg, DC** (www.drberg.com).

A ketogenic diet consists of high quality fats, moderate protein and low carbohydrates.

Q&A

Should you pay attention more to Net Carbs or Total Carbs on a Keto diet?

- It's a personal preference. Net Carbs are the result of subtracting the Fiber content from the Total Carbohydrates and any Sugar Alcohols (if any are present), eg. erythritol, sorbitol, and xylitol.
- Some people desire to focus on limiting Total Carbs and others, limiting just Net Carbs. Since fiber is important in the diet, if you focus on the Net Carbs, it should ensure that you're getting fiber in your diet.

How Many Net Carbs Should You Eat In a Day?

- Keep to less than 20 grams of net carbs per day for optimal weight loss
- Mid range: 20-50 grams of net carbs per day
- Max: 50-100 grams of net carbs per day

- Broccoli
- Cauliflower
- Kale
- Leafy greens
- Asparagus
- Avocado
- Macadamia nuts
- Pumpkin seeds
- Raspberries

- Extra Virgin Olive Oil
- Coconut Oil
- Avocados and Avocado Oil
- Flaxseed and Chia Seeds
- Nuts & Nut Butters
- Ghee and Organic Butter

Sample Keto Meals & Snacks... Plus Tips

Sample Keto Breakfasts

- Eggs, cooked any way you like; with or without cheese and veggies (many egg recipes can be poured into muffin pans and put in the freezer to have as snacks throughout the day)
- Bacon
- Sausage
- Keto Waffles (see recipe, pg 67)
- Keto Breakfast Tacos (see recipe, pg 65)
- Keto Pancakes (see recipe, pg 66)
- Cinnamon Roll Keto 'Oatmeal' (see recipe, pg 59)
- Pea Protein Shake (purchase in store or online - check for carb count)
- Whey Protein Shake (purchase in store or online - check for carb count)

Sample Keto Snacks

- Homemade guacamole with pork rinds (or kale chips that are homemade or store bought)
- Artichoke dip with kale chips
- Avocados (filling and satisfying)
- Olives
- Almond butter on low carb cracker or vegetable
- Beef jerky
- Nuts (relatively low in carbs if limited)
- Berries (relatively low in carbs if limited)
- Raspberry Lemon Popsicles (see recipe, pg 61)
- Low Carb Chocolate Chip Cookies (see recipe, pg 55)
- All cheeses

- Salads
- Tuna or chicken salad w/mayo; add some cucumber or celery (eat alone or in a lettuce wrap or low carb tortilla wrap)
- Salmon patties made with wild alaskan salmon; fresh or canned (if canned, mix salmon with egg and fry up in a pan)
- Burger and veggies without the bun; add slices of avocado
- Cauliflower crust frozen pizzas (look for low carb varieties; some are high in carbs)
- Stews and casseroles; add bone broth for juice and any meat and veggies

- Cook things in or with coconut oil, olive oil, organic butter, or ghee butter.
- Add flax seed, coconut oil, or chia seeds to smoothies and salads.
- If sweetness is desired in a recipe, smoothie or drink, substitute with Stevia
- Use a Spiralizer with zucchini or squash to replace pasta in recipes.
- Stay away from soda -- instead, drink hot or iced tea; hot or iced coffee; protein shakes; Glaceau Vitamin Zero Water or Bai Water (purchase in store or online); lemonade made with water and real lemon (juiced) and no sugar unless Stevia.
- Alcohol -- stick with spirits vs. wine or beer

NUTRITION FACTS

FACTS

categorized

Vegetables	Serving Size	Total Carbs (g)	Net Carbs (g)	Fiber (g)	Sugar (g)	Total Fat (g)	Sat Fat (g)	Protein (g)	Sodium (mg)	Calories
Alfalfa Sprouts, raw	1 c	1	0	1	0	0	0	1	2	8
Artichokes, fresh, boiled, single	1	14	7	7	1	0	0	4	72	64
Artichokes, raw, single	1	14	1	13	1	0	0	4	120	60
Arugula, raw	1 c	1	0	1	0	0	0	1	5	5
Asparagus, fresh or frozen, boiled	1 c	7	3	4	2	0	0	4	25	40
Asparagus, raw, single spear	1	1	1	0	0	0	0	0	0	3
Bamboo shoots, raw	1/2 c	4	2	2	2	0	0	2	3	21
Bean sprouts, mung, raw	1 c	6	4	2	2	0	0	3	6	31
Beans, green snap, fresh, cooked	1 c	10	6	4	5	0	0	2	1	44
Beans, green snap, raw, single	1	0	0	0	0	0	0	0	0	2
Beets, fresh, boiled	1 c	16	13	3	13	0	0	3	121	69
Beets, raw, single	1	8	6	2	6	0	0	1	64	35
Bok Choy, shredded	1 c	2	1	1	1	0	0	1	46	9
Broccoli, fresh, boiled, chopped	1 c	11	6	5	2	1	0	4	64	55
Broccoli, raw, chopped	1 c	6	4	2	2	0	0	3	30	31
Broccoli, raw, single flower	1	1	1	0	0	0	0	0	4	4
Brussel Sprouts, fresh, boiled, whole	1 c	11	7	4	3	1	0	4	33	56
Brussel Sprouts, raw, pieces	1 tbsp	1	1	0	0	0	0	0	1	2
Cabbage, green, fresh, cooked	1 c	8	5	3	4	0	0	2	12	35
Cabbage, green, raw, chopped	1 c	5	3	2	3	0	0	1	16	22
Cabbage, red, fresh, cooked	1 c	10	6	4	5	0	0	2	42	44
Cabbage, red, raw, chopped	1 c	7	5	2	3	0	0	1	24	28
Carrots, baby, raw, single	1	1	1	0	1	0	0	0	8	4
Carrots, fresh, cooked, diced	1 c	12	8	4	5	0	0	1	84	51
Carrots, fresh, single	1	6	4	2	3	0	0	1	42	25
Cauliflower, fresh, boiled	1 c	5	2	3	3	0	0	2	19	29
Cauliflower, raw, single flower	1	1	1	0	0	0	0	0	4	3
Celery, fresh, cooked	1 c	6	4	2	4	0	0	1	137	27
Celery, raw, single stalk	1	1	0	1	1	0	0	0	32	6
Cilantro, raw, single sprig	1	0	0	0	0	0	0	0	1	1

Vegetables (cont')	Serving Size	Total Carbs (g)	Net Carbs (g)	Fiber (g)	Sugar (g)	Total Fat (g)	Sat Fat (g)	Protein (g)	Sodium (mg)	Calories
Collards, fresh, cooked	1 c	11	8	3	1	1	0	5	29	63
Corn, canned, cream	1 c	46	43	3	8	1	0	5	668	184
Corn, canned, whole	1 c	24	21	3	7	2	0	4	336	110
Corn, single ear, cooked	1	22	19	3	5	2	0	4	1	99
Corn, single ear, raw	1	17	15	2	3	1	0	3	14	77
Corn, frozen, whole kernel	1 c	32	28	4	5	1	0	4	2	134
Cucumber, raw, single slice	1	0	0	0	0	0	0	0	0	1
Edamame, fresh, cooked	1 c	20	12	8	3	12	1	22	25	254
Eggplant, fresh, cooked	1 c	9	6	3	3	0	0	1	1	35
Eggplant, raw, peeled, single	1	27	13	14	16	1	0	5	9	115
Fennel, raw, sliced	1 c	6	3	3	3	0	0	1	45	27
Garlic, raw, single clove	1	1	1	0	0	0	0	0	1	5
Jicama, cooked	1 c	12	5	7	2	0	0	1	5	51
Jicama, raw, sliced	1 c	3	1	2	1	0	0	0	2	14
Kale, fresh, cooked	1 c	7	4	3	2	0	0	3	30	36
Kale, raw	1 c	1	0	1	0	0	0	1	6	8
Leeks, fresh, cooked, single	1	9	8	1	3	0	0	1	12	38
Leeks, raw, single	1	13	11	2	4	0	0	1	18	54
Lettuce, Boston, Bib, Butterhead	1 c	1	0	1	1	0	0	1	3	7
Lettuce, Iceberg	1 c	2	1	1	1	0	0	1	6	8
Lettuce, Romaine	1 c	2	1	1	1	0	0	1	4	8
Mushrooms, canned	1 c	8	4	4	4	1	0	3	663	39
Mushrooms, fresh, cooked	1 c	8	5	3	4	1	0	3	3	44
Mushrooms, raw, single	1	1	1	0	0	0	0	1	1	4
Mustard Greens, fresh, cooked	1 c	6	3	3	2	1	0	4	13	36
Okra, fresh, cooked	1 c	7	3	4	3	0	0	3	10	35
Olives, black, raw, single	1	0	0	0	0	0	0	0	29	5
Olives, green, raw, single	1	0	0	0	0	1	0	0	53	5
Onions, green (scallions), tops & bulb, single	1	1	1	0	1	0	0	0	2	5
Onions, white, yellow, red, fresh, cooked	1 c	13	11	2	6	0	0	2	4	56

Vegetables (cont')	Serving Size	Total Carbs (g)	Net Carbs (g)	Fiber (g)	Sugar (g)	Total Fat (g)	Sat Fat (g)	Protein (g)	Sodium (mg)	Calories
Onions, white, yellow, red, raw, single	1	10	8	2	5	0	0	1	4	44
Parsley, raw	1 tbsp	0	0	0	0	0	0	0	2	1
Parsnip, cooked, single	1	17	4	3	5	0	0	1	10	70
Peas, green, canned	1 c	20	11	9	5	1	0	8	478	119
Peas, green, fresh or frozen, cooked	1 c	23	16	7	7	0	0	8	115	125
Peas, snowpeas, raw, single pod	1	0	0	0	0	0	0	0	0	1
Pepper, jalapeno, canned	1 oz	2	2	0	1	0	0	1	25	10
Pepper, jalapeno, raw, single	1	1	1	0	1	0	0	0	0	4
Pepper, sweet, fresh, cooked, chopped	1 c	9	8	1	7	0	0	1	3	38
Pepper, sweet, raw, single	1	7	4	3	5	0	0	1	5	37
Potato, baked, skin not eaten, single	1	28	26	2	2	0	0	3	7	122
Potato, boiled w/o skin, single	1	33	30	3	2	0	0	3	8	144
Potato, french fries, baked, steak, single	1	2	2	0	0	1	0	0	29	14
Potato, french fries, fried, single	1 c	43	39	4	2	15	2	4	218	319
Potato, hashbrowns	1 c	15	13	2	1	0	0	2	25	70
Potato, mashed	1 c	44	40	4	3	9	2	4	359	268
Potato, sweet (yam), baked, single	1	24	20	4	7	0	0	2	41	103
Radish, raw, single	1	0	0	0	0	0	0	0	2	1
Seaweed, dulse, dried	1 oz	7	6	1	0	1	0	10	85	62
Seaweed, spirulina, raw	1 oz	1	1	0	0	0	0	2	28	7
Spinach, canned	1 c	7	2	5	1	1	0	6	420	49
Spinach, frozen, cooked	1 c	9	2	7	1	2	0	8	184	65
Spinach, raw	1 c	1	0	1	0	0	0	1	24	7
Squash, butternut, baked	1 c	22	15	7	4	0	0	2	8	82
Squash, spaghetti, baked	1 c	10	8	2	4	0	0	1	28	42
Tomato, canned	1 c	8	3	5	6	1	0	2	276	38
Tomato, cherry, single	1	1	1	0	0	0	0	0	1	3
Tomato, fresh, cooked	1 c	10	8	2	6	0	0	2	26	43
Tomato, raw, single	1	5	3	2	3	0	0	1	6	22
Tomato, sundried, jar w/oil	3 pcs	4	2	2	3	1	0	1	220	30

Vegetables (cont')	Serving Size	Total Carbs (g)	Net Carbs (g)	Fiber (g)	Sugar (g)	Total Fat (g)	Sat Fat (g)	Protein (g)	Sodium (mg)	Calories
Turnip, fresh, cooked, single	1	6	4	2	4	0	0	1	19	26
Turnip, raw, single	1	8	6	2	5	0	0	1	82	34
Watercress, raw	1 c	0	0	0	0	0	0	1	14	4
Zucchini, fresh, cooked	1 c	6	4	2	4	1	0	2	6	32
Zucchini, raw, single	1	6	4	2	5	1	0	2	16	33

Eggs, Milk & Cream	Serving Size	Total Carbs (g)	Net Carbs (g)	Fiber (g)	Sugar (g)	Total Fat (g)	Sat Fat (g)	Protein (g)	Sodium (mg)	Calories
Cream, coffee, powdered	1 tsp	1	1	0	0	1	0	0	2	10
Cream, half and half	1 tbsp	1	1	0	1	2	1	1	9	19
Cream, sour	1 tbsp	1	1	0	1	3	2	0	4	29
Cream, whipping, heavy	1 fl oz	1	1	0	1	11	7	1	8	101
Egg, substitute, white, single	1	0	0	0	0	0	0	5	171	24
Egg, white, cooked, single	1	0	0	0	0	0	0	4	55	17
Egg, whole, raw or cooked, single	1	1	1	0	1	5	2	6	62	78
Egg, yolk, cooked, single	1	1	1	0	0	4	2	3	8	54
Milk, almond, plain, unsweetened	1 c	1	1	0	0	3	0	1	170	36
Milk, buttermilk, whole	1 c	12	12	0	12	8	5	8	257	152
Milk, cashew, plain, unsweetened	1 c	1	1	0	0	2	0	1	160	25
Milk, chocolate, whole	1 c	26	24	2	24	9	5	8	150	208
Milk, cow, 2%	1 c	12	12	0	12	5	3	8	115	122
Milk, cow, whole	1 c	12	12	0	12	8	5	8	105	149
Milk, goat	1 c	11	11	0	11	10	7	9	122	169
Milk, rice, plain, unsweetened	1 c	7	4	3	2	3	0	0	135	52
Milk, soy, plain, unsweetened	1 c	4	1	3	1	4	1	8	85	74

Yogurt & Cheese	Serving Size	Total Carbs (g)	Net Carbs (g)	Fiber (g)	Sugar (g)	Total Fat (g)	Sat Fat (g)	Protein (g)	Sodium (mg)	Calories
Cheese, american, single slice	1	1	1	0	0	6	3	3	316	69
Cheese, blue, crumbled	1 tbsp	0	0	0	0	2	2	2	97	30
Cheese, brick, single cracker slice	1	0	0	0	0	3	2	2	50	33
Cheese, brie	1 tbsp	0	0	0	0	4	3	3	94	50
Cheese, cheddar, single cracker slice	1	0	0	0	0	3	2	2	59	36
Cheese, cheddar, shredded	1 c	4	4	0	1	38	21	26	738	457
Cheese, colby, single slice	1	1	1	0	0	9	6	7	169	110
Cheese, cottage, 2%	1 c	11	11	0	9	5	3	24	696	183
Cheese, cottage, whole	1 c	7	7	0	6	9	4	23	764	206
Cheese, cream	1 c	7	7	0	6	9	4	23	764	206
Cheese, edam, single cracker slice	1	0	0	0	0	7	5	7	270	89
Cheese, feta, crumbled	1 tbsp	0	0	0	0	2	1	1	86	25
Cheese, goat, soft, crumbled	1 tbsp	0	0	0	0	2	1	2	40	23
Cheese, gouda, single cracker slice	1	0	0	0	0	3	2	2	74	32
Cheese, gruyere, single cracker slice	1	0	0	0	0	3	2	3	64	37
Cheese, mozzerella, part skim, shredded	1 c	6	6	0	2	22	13	27	753	333
Cheese, parmesan, fresh or dry, grated	1 tbsp	1	1	0	0	2	1	2	102	27
Cheese, ricotta, part skim	1 c	13	13	0	1	20	12	28	243	340
Cheese, ricotta, whole	1 c	8	8	0	5	32	20	28	207	428
Cheese, romano, fresh or dry, grated	1 tbsp	1	1	0	0	2	1	2	113	26
Cheese, swiss, single slice	1	0	0	0	0	7	4	6	39	83
Kefir, lowfat, flavored	8 fl oz	20	20	0	20	2	2	11	125	139
Kefir, whole, plain	8 fl oz	11	11	0	10	8	5	12	130	160
Yogurt, greek, nonfat, plain	6 oz	6	6	0	6	1	0	17	61	100
Yogurt, lowfat, flavored	6 oz	34	33	1	27	3	2	5	67	180
Yogurt, lowfat, plain	1 c	17	17	0	17	4	3	13	172	154
Yogurt, plain, whole	1 c	11	11	0	11	8	5	9	113	150

Oils, Butters, Dressings & Spreads	Serving Size	Total Carbs (g)	Net Carbs (g)	Fiber (g)	Sugar (g)	Total Fat (g)	Sat Fat (g)	Protein (g)	Sodium (mg)	Calories
Butter, almond, unsalted	1 tbsp	3	1	2	1	9	1	3	1	96
Butter, cashew, unsalted	1 tbsp	4	4	0	1	8	2	3	2	94
Butter, ghee	1 tbsp	0	0	0	0	8	8	0	0	112
Butter, margarine	1 tbsp	0	0	0	0	11	2	0	93	99
Butter, peanut, organic, no stir	1 tbsp	2	0	2	1	9	1	3	33	100
Butter, raw, salted	1 tbsp	0	0	0	0	12	7	0	0	102
Butter, sunflower seed	1 tbsp	4	3	1	2	9	1	3	1	99
Butter, tahini, sesame seed butter	1 tbsp	3	2	1	0	8	1	3	17	89
Dressing, blue cheese	1 tbsp	1	1	0	1	8	1	0	98	74
Dressing, caesar	1 tbsp	1	1	0	0	9	1	0	178	77
Dressing, creamy ranch	1 tbsp	0	0	0	0	7	1	0	210	61
Dressing, Italian	1 tbsp	2	2	0	2	3	0	0	146	35
Dressing, oil vinaigrette	1 tbsp	0	0	0	0	9	1	0	197	82
Jelly, grape, squeezable	1 tbsp	13	13	0	12	0	0	0	5	50
Lard (made from animal fats)	1 tbsp	0	0	0	0	13	5	0	0	116
Nutella	1 tbsp	12	11	1	10	6	1	1	8	100
Oil, canola	1 tbsp	0	0	0	0	14	1	0	0	120
Oil, coconut	1 tbsp	0	0	0	0	14	11	0	0	122
Oil, corn	1 tbsp	0	0	0	0	14	2	0	0	123
Oil, flaxseed	1 tbsp	0	0	0	0	14	1	0	0	120
Oil, olive, extra virgin, cold pressed	1 tbsp	0	0	0	0	14	2	0	0	119
Oil, peanut	1 tbsp	0	0	0	0	14	2	0	0	120
Oil, safflower	1 tbsp	0	0	0	0	14	1	0	0	120
Oil, sesame	1 tbsp	0	0	0	0	14	2	0	0	120
Oil, sunflower	1 tbsp	0	0	0	0	14	1	0	0	120
Oil, vegetable	1 tbsp	0	0	0	0	14	2	0	0	120
Oil, walnut	1 tbsp	0	0	0	0	14	1	0	0	120

Meat & Poultry	Serving Size	Total Carbs (g)	Net Carbs (g)	Fiber (g)	Sugar (g)	Total Fat (g)	Sat Fat (g)	Protein (g)	Sodium (mg)	Calories
Bison, steak, 3 oz	1	0	0	0	0	11	5	54	103	332
Chicken, breast, baked or roasted, 1/2 breast	1	0	0	0	0	8	2	29	70	193
Chicken, cornish game hen, roasted, 3 oz	1	0	0	0	0	16	4	19	54	220
Chicken, leg, breaded and fried	1	3	3	0	0	16	4	30	99	285
Chicken, whole, roasted, 3 oz	1	0	0	0	0	12	3	23	530	210
Flank, steak, 3 oz	1	0	0	0	0	7	3	24	48	165
Ground beef, 85% lean	1 c	0	0	0	0	31	12	56	139	520
Pork, chops, single	1	0	0	0	0	7	2	46	105	256
Pork, ground	1 c	0	0	0	0	46	16	59	193	652
Pork, loin, 3 oz	1	0	0	0	0	3	1	22	49	122
Pork, ribs, spare, single	1	0	0	0	0	11	4	10	33	139
Rib roast, 3 oz	1	0	0	0	0	20	9	20	43	258
Ribeye, 4 oz	1	0	0	0	0	12	6	21	60	190
Round roast, 3 oz	1	0	0	0	0	9	3	24	32	180
Rump roast, 4 oz	1	0	0	0	0	14	5	23	60	220
Short ribs, 3 oz	1	0	0	0	0	13	4	25	64	213
Sirloin, 3 oz	1	0	0	0	0	8	3	25	52	180
Stew beef, cubed	1 c	0	0	0	0	20	8	36	77	335
T-bone, 4 oz	1	0	0	0	0	19	8	21	60	260
Tenderloin, 3 oz	1	0	0	0	0	15	6	23	46	227
Turkey, ground	1 c	0	0	0	0	40	11	58	196	596
Turkey, whole, roasted, 3 oz	1	0	0	0	0	6	2	24	88	161
Veal, cutlets, 3 oz	1	0	0	0	0	2	1	27	75	128
Veal, ground	1 c	0	0	0	0	13	5	57	197	355
Venison, stew meat	1 c	0	0	0	0	8	3	74	133	388

Fish & Shell Fish	Serving Size	Total Carbs (g)	Net Carbs (g)	Fiber (g)	Sugar (g)	Total Fat (g)	Sat Fat (g)	Protein (g)	Sodium (mg)	Calories
Anchovies, canned, pieces	6	0	0	0	0	3	0	4	970	40
Bass, 3 oz fillet	1	0	0	0	0	3	1	15	56	91
Calamari, squid, breaded	1 c	18	17	1	1	16	3	23	518	315

17

Fish & Shell Fish (cont')	Serving Size	Total Carbs (g)	Net Carbs (g)	Fiber (g)	Sugar (g)	Total Fat (g)	Sat Fat (g)	Protein (g)	Sodium (mg)	Calories
Catfish, 6 oz fillet	1	0	0	0	0	10	2	26	170	206
Caviar	1 tsp	0	0	0	0	1	0	1	80	14
Clams, fresh, cooked, single	1	0	0	0	0	0	0	3	14	18
Cod, 4 oz fillet	1	0	0	0	0	0	0	18	121	76
Crab leg, single	1	0	0	0	0	0	0	8	168	35
Crab meat	3 oz	0	0	0	0	1	0	19	320	90
Crayfish or crawfish	1 c	0	0	0	0	3	0	41	231	201
Fish sticks, single stick	1	3	3	0	1	2	0	2	52	36
Haddock, 7 oz fillet	1	0	0	0	0	1	0	30	392	135
Halibut, 14 oz	1	0	0	0	0	5	1	72	261	353
Herring, 7 oz fillet	1	0	0	0	0	26	6	30	137	360
Lobster, 1 lb	1	0	0	0	0	1	0	22	574	105
Mackerel, 8 oz fillet	1	0	0	0	0	18	5	45	194	354
Oysters, canned, 8 oz	1	1	1	0	0	5	1	15	234	142
Oysters, fresh, cooked	1 c	2	2	0	0	11	3	46	520	400
Perch, 2 oz fillet	1	0	0	0	0	1	0	9	174	48
Pike, 14 oz fillet	1	0	0	0	0	3	1	77	152	350
Salmon, wild alaskan, canned	1/4 c	0	0	0	0	7	2	13	230	110
Salmon, wild alaskan, fresh	6 oz	0	0	0	0	10	2	36	190	230
Sardines, canned, water, 4 oz	1	0	0	0	0	9	3	21	118	164
Scallops	1 c	13	13	0	0	2	1	50	1637	272
Shrimp, breaded	1 c	31	30	1	3	17	3	15	737	335
Shrimp, frozen	1 c	2	2	0	0	3	1	33	1373	173
Smelt	1 c	0	0	0	0	8	1	56	189	304
Snapper, 8 oz fillet	1	0	0	0	0	3	1	45	97	218
Trout, rainbow, 3 oz fillet	1	0	0	0	0	5	1	17	43	119
Tuna, steaks, 5 oz	1	0	0	0	0	1	0	17	25	75
Tuna, white, canned, 5 oz	1	0	0	0	0	4	1	31	65	165
Walleye, 6 oz fillet	1	0	0	0	0	2	0	30	81	148
Whitefish, 7 oz fillet	1	0	0	0	0	12	2	38	100	265

Processed Meats	Serving Size	Total Carbs (g)	Net Carbs (g)	Fiber (g)	Sugar (g)	Total Fat (g)	Sat Fat (g)	Protein (g)	Sodium (mg)	Calories
Bacon, single slice	1	0	0	0	0	3	1	3	135	37
Bologna, single slice	1	2	2	0	0	8	3	3	299	95
Chicken, canned, 5 oz	1	2	2	0	0	2	1	23	500	127
Corned Beef, single slice	1	0	0	0	0	1	1	4	281	30
Deli Meat, turkey, single slice	1	0	0	0	0	0	0	4	206	21
Ham, honey roasted, 2 oz	1	4	4	0	4	3	1	10	540	80
Pastrami, beef, single slice	1	0	0	0	0	2	1	6	379	41
Salami, pork and beef, single slice	1	0	0	0	0	5	2	4	209	57
Sausage, bratwurst, single link	1	2	2	0	2	28	8	8	698	230
Sausage, breakfast, single patty	1	0	0	0	0	15	5	5	347	153
Sausage, italian, single link	1	3	3	0	1	21	7	14	557	258
Sausage, liver, liverwurst, single slice	1	0	0	0	0	5	2	3	155	59
Sausage, polish kielbasa, single link	1	2	2	0	2	20	7	8	670	221
Sausage, summer, beef, single slice	1	0	0	0	0	6	3	3	328	71
Sausage, vienna, single link	1	0	0	0	0	3	1	2	141	38
Weiner, hot dog, single link	1	1	0	1	1	13	4	7	530	140

Legumes, Nuts & Seeds	Serving Size	Total Carbs (g)	Net Carbs (g)	Fiber (g)	Sugar (g)	Total Fat (g)	Sat Fat (g)	Protein (g)	Sodium (mg)	Calories
Beans, black, canned, drained	1 c	45	27	18	1	1	0	14	662	241
Beans, black, dry, cooked	1 c	41	26	15	1	1	0	15	2	227
Beans, garbanzo (chick peas), canned, drained	1 c	37	26	11	7	5	0	12	403	228
Beans, garbanzo (chick peas), dry, cooked	1 c	45	32	13	8	4	0	15	12	269
Beans, kidney, canned, drained	1 c	38	28	10	7	2	0	14	409	220
Beans, kidney, dry, cooked	1 c	40	29	11	1	1	0	15	2	225
Beans, lentils, canned, drained	1 c	40	28	12	1	1	0	18	471	230
Beans, lentils, dry, cooked	1 c	40	28	12	1	1	0	18	4	230
Beans, navy, canned, drained	1 c	47	28	19	1	1	0	15	701	255
Beans, navy, dry, cooked	1 c	47	28	19	1	1	0	15	0	255

Legumes, Nuts & Seeds (cont')	Serving Size	Total Carbs (g)	Net Carbs (g)	Fiber (g)	Sugar (g)	Total Fat (g)	Sat Fat (g)	Protein (g)	Sodium (mg)	Calories
Beans, pinto, canned, drained	1 c	35	25	10	1	2	0	12	409	195
Beans, pinto, dry, cooked	1 c	45	30	15	1	1	0	15	2	245
Beans, white, canned, drained	1 c	56	43	13	1	1	0	19	891	299
Beans, white, dry, cooked	1 c	48	35	13	1	1	0	18	11	263
Nuts, almonds, raw, unsalted, single	3	1	0	1	0	2	0	0	0	21
Nuts, brazils, raw, unsalted, single	3	2	1	1	0	10	2	2	0	93
Nuts, cashews, raw, unsalted, single	3	2	2	0	0	2	0	1	0	27
Nuts, hazelnuts, single	3	1	1	0	0	3	0	1	0	26
Nuts, macadamia, single	3	1	0	1	0	6	1	1	0	56
Nuts, mixed nuts, dry, roasted, salted, single	3	1	1	0	0	2	0	1	15	26
Nuts, peanuts, single	3	0	0	0	0	1	0	1	1	15
Nuts, pecans, single	3	1	0	1	0	6	1	1	0	62
Nuts, pine nuts	1 tbsp	2	1	1	1	5	1	1	6	53
Nuts, pistachios, single	3	1	1	0	0	1	0	0	0	10
Nuts, walnuts, single halves	3	1	1	0	0	4	0	1	0	37
Seeds, chia	1 tbsp	4	1	3	0	3	0	2	2	49
Seeds, flaxseed, raw	1 tbsp	2	0	2	0	3	0	1	2	37
Seeds, pumpkin, raw, unsalted	1/4 c	4	2	2	0	13	3	11	0	180
Seeds, sunflower	1/4 c	7	4	3	1	18	2	7	3	204
Tempeh, single patty	1	17	9	8	6	25	6	46	20	436
Tofu, single slice	1	2	2	0	1	2	0	6	30	52

Fruit & Fruit Juices	Serving Size	Total Carbs (g)	Net Carbs (g)	Fiber (g)	Sugar (g)	Total Fat (g)	Sat Fat (g)	Protein (g)	Sodium (mg)	Calories
Apple, juice or cider, unsweetened	1 c	28	27	1	24	0	0	0	10	114
Apple, raw, w/o skin, single	1	21	19	2	16	0	0	0	0	77
Apple, raw, w/skin, single	1	25	21	4	19	0	0	1	2	95
Apricots, dried	1 tbsp	5	4	1	4	0	0	0	1	20
Apricots, raw, single	1	4	3	1	3	0	0	1	0	17
Avocado, black, single	1	12	3	9	0	21	3	3	11	227

Fruit & Fruit Juices (cont')	Serving Size	Total Carbs (g)	Net Carbs (g)	Fiber (g)	Sugar (g)	Total Fat (g)	Sat Fat (g)	Protein (g)	Sodium (mg)	Calories
Banana, raw, single	1	27	24	3	14	0	0	1	1	105
Blackberries, frozen	1 c	24	16	8	16	1	0	2	2	97
Blackberries, raw, single	1	1	1	0	0	0	0	0	0	2
Blueberries, frozen	1 c	28	22	6	19	2	0	1	2	117
Blueberries, raw, single	1	0	0	0	0	0	0	0	0	1
Cherries, frozen	1 c	22	19	3	18	0	0	2	0	88
Cherries, sweet, pitted, single	1	1	1	0	1	0	0	0	0	5
Clementine, single	1	9	8	1	7	0	0	1	1	35
Coconut, milk, canned, unsweetened	1 fl oz	1	1	0	1	4	4	0	10	46
Coconut, water	1 fl oz	1	1	0	1	0	0	0	0	6
Coconut, whole, single	1	61	25	36	25	133	118	13	80	1405
Cranberries, dried, sweetened	1 tbsp	24	22	2	21	0	0	0	1	87
Cranberry, juice, unsweetened	1 fl oz	4	4	0	3	0	0	0	1	13
Dates, pitted, medjool, single	1	18	16	2	16	0	0	0	0	67
Figs, dried, single	1	5	4	1	4	0	0	0	1	21
Figs, raw, single	1	8	7	1	7	0	0	0	0	30
Grape, juice, unsweetened	1 fl oz	5	5	0	5	0	0	0	2	19
Grapefruit, juice	1 fl oz	3	3	0	2	0	0	0	0	12
Grapefruit, raw, single	1	27	23	4	18	0	0	2	0	108
Grapes, raw, seedless, single	1	1	1	0	1	0	0	0	0	3
Kiwi, raw, single	1	10	8	2	6	0	0	1	2	42
Lemon, juice	1 tbsp	1	1	0	0	0	0	0	0	3
Lemon, raw, single	1	4	3	1	1	0	0	0	1	12
Lime, raw, single	1	7	5	2	1	0	0	1	1	20
Mango, raw, single	1	50	45	5	46	1	0	3	3	202
Melon, cantaloupe, cubed	1 c	13	12	1	13	0	0	1	26	54
Melon, honeydew, cubed	1 c	17	15	2	16	0	0	1	34	69
Melon, watermelon, cubed	1 c	12	11	1	9	0	0	1	2	46
Nectarine, raw, single	1	15	13	2	11	1	0	2	0	63

21

Fruit & Fruit Juices (cont')	Serving Size	Total Carbs (g)	Net Carbs (g)	Fiber (g)	Sugar (g)	Total Fat (g)	Sat Fat (g)	Protein (g)	Sodium (mg)	Calories
Orange, juice	1 fl oz	3	3	0	3	0	0	0	0	14
Orange, raw, single	1	15	12	3	12	0	0	1	0	62
Papaya, raw, single	1	33	28	5	24	1	0	1	24	131
Peach, raw, single	1	14	12	2	13	0	0	1	0	59
Pear, raw, single	1	27	21	6	17	0	0	1	0	102
Pineapple, juice	1 fl oz	4	4	0	3	0	0	0	1	17
Pineapple, raw, chunks	1 c	22	20	2	16	0	0	1	2	83
Plantain, raw, single	1	57	53	4	27	1	0	2	7	218
Plum, raw, single	1	6	5	1	6	0	0	0	0	25
Pomegranate, raw, single	1	53	42	11	39	3	0	5	9	234
Prune, juice, unsweetened	1 fl oz	6	6	0	5	0	0	0	1	23
Prunes, dried	1 tbsp	7	6	1	4	0	0	0	0	26
Raisins, uncooked	1 tbsp	7	7	0	5	0	0	0	1	27
Raspberries, raw, single	1	0	0	0	0	0	0	0	0	1
Rhubarb, cooked, unsweetened	1 c	5	2	3	2	0	0	2	2	17
Rhubarb, raw, stalk	1	2	1	1	1	0	0	1	2	11
Strawberries, frozen, unsweetened	1 c	20	15	5	10	0	0	1	4	77
Strawberries, raw, single	1	1	1	0	1	0	0	0	0	4
Tangerine (mandarin), raw, single	1	12	10	2	9	0	0	1	2	47

Breads & Grains	Serving Size	Total Carbs (g)	Net Carbs (g)	Fiber (g)	Sugar (g)	Total Fat (g)	Sat Fat (g)	Protein (g)	Sodium (mg)	Calories
Bagel, plain, single	1	52	50	2	7	2	1	10	460	270
Barley, pearled, cooked	1 c	43	34	9	1	1	0	5	83	193
Biscuit, homemade, single	1	16	15	1	1	8	2	2	164	149
Bread, wheat, single slice	2	38	32	6	6	3	0	8	300	200
Bread, white, gluten free, single slice	2	18	14	4	4	2	0	2	210	170
Bread, white, single slice	2	29	27	2	5	2	0	4	180	140
Bread, zero carb, single slice	1	7	0	7	0	2	1	7	90	45

Breads & Grains (cont')	Serving Size	Total Carbs (g)	Net Carbs (g)	Fiber (g)	Sugar (g)	Total Fat (g)	Sat Fat (g)	Protein (g)	Sodium (mg)	Calories
Croissant Roll, single	1	27	26	1	4	15	9	5	75	260
Croutons, seasoned, 1 svg of 7g	1	4	3	1	0	1	0	1	76	33
Dinner Roll, sweet, single	1	16	15	1	5	2	1	3	76	96
Dinner Roll, wheat, single	1	13	12	1	1	2	1	2	147	76
English Muffin, wheat, single whole	1	27	23	4	5	1	0	6	240	134
English Muffin, white, single whole	1	25	23	2	2	1	0	5	242	129
French Toast, white, homemade, single	1	15	14	1	3	5	1	5	184	125
Hamburger/Hot Dog Bun, wheat, single	1	18	15	3	2	2	0	5	196	108
Hamburger/Hot Dog Bun, white, single	1	22	21	1	3	2	0	4	212	120
Oatmeal, cooked	1 c	55	47	8	1	5	1	11	5	307
Pancake, homemade, single	1	13	13	0	3	4	1	3	306	99
Pasta Noodles, cooked	1 c	43	40	3	1	1	0	8	1	221
Pita, white, single	1	33	32	1	0	1	0	6	322	165
Pita, whole grain, single	1	32	28	4	2	1	0	6	300	149
Quinoa, cooked	1 c	39	34	5	2	4	0	8	13	222
Rice, brown, cooked	1 c	52	49	3	1	2	1	6	8	249
Rice, white, cooked	1 c	45	44	1	0	0	0	4	2	205
Tortilla, corn, single	1	11	10	1	0	1	0	1	11	52
Tortilla, flour, single	1	26	25	1	1	3	1	4	400	140
Waffle, homemade, single	1	31	30	1	5	17	5	7	461	299
Waffle, plain, frozen, single	1	15	14	1	2	3	1	2	223	100

Sauces, Dips & Sides	Serving Size	Total Carbs (g)	Net Carbs (g)	Fiber (g)	Sugar (g)	Total Fat (g)	Sat Fat (g)	Protein (g)	Sodium (mg)	Calories
BBQ sauce, homemade	1 tbsp	4	4	0	3	0	0	0	99	15
Coleslaw	1 c	12	9	3	8	37	6	2	344	384
Guacamole	1 tbsp	1	0	1	0	1	0	0	59	14
Horseradish	1 tbsp	2	1	1	1	0	0	0	63	7
Hot Pepper Sauce	1 tsp	0	0	0	0	0	0	0	124	1
Hummus	1 tbsp	3	2	1	1	1	0	1	66	27

Sauces, Dips & Sides (cont')	Serving Size	Total Carbs (g)	Net Carbs (g)	Fiber (g)	Sugar (g)	Total Fat (g)	Sat Fat (g)	Protein (g)	Sodium (mg)	Calories
Ketchup (Catsup)	1 tbsp	4	4	0	3	0	0	0	136	15
Mayonnaise	1 tbsp	0	0	0	0	10	2	0	87	94
Miso	1 tbsp	4	3	1	1	1	0	2	641	34
Mustard, sauce	1 tbsp	1	0	1	0	1	0	1	172	9
Onion Dip	1 tbsp	2	2	0	1	2	2	1	105	30
Pesto, homemade	1 tbsp	1	1	0	0	8	2	1	57	79
Pickle, single slice	1	0	0	0	0	0	0	0	169	2
Pickle, sour, single whole	1	2	1	1	1	0	0	0	785	8
Potato Salad, homemade	1 c	28	25	3	0	21	4	7	1323	358
Relish, sweet pickle	1 tsp	2	2	0	2	0	0	0	41	7
Salsa	1 tbsp	1	1	0	1	0	0	0	115	5
Sauce, soy	1 tbsp	1	1	0	0	0	0	1	875	8
Sauce, spaghetti, homemade	1 c	15	10	5	9	10	2	3	927	146
Sauce, tartar	1 tbsp	1	1	0	0	10	2	0	145	95
Sauce, tomato	1 c	13	9	4	9	1	0	3	1161	59
Sauce, worcheshire	1 tsp	1	1	0	1	0	0	0	56	5
Sauerkraut	1 c	10	3	7	3	0	0	2	1560	45
Syrup, maple, organic	1 tbsp	13	13	0	13	0	0	0	2	50
Syrup, pancake	1 tbsp	14	14	0	8	0	0	0	12	51

Baking Ingredients & Sweeteners	Serving Size	Total Carbs (g)	Net Carbs (g)	Fiber (g)	Sugar (g)	Total Fat (g)	Sat Fat (g)	Protein (g)	Sodium (mg)	Calories
Baking powder	1 tbsp	4	4	0	0	0	0	0	1463	7
Baking soda	1 tsp	0	0	0	0	0	0	0	1259	0
Black Pepper, ground	1 tsp	2	1	1	0	0	0	0	1	6
Bread crumbs, plain	1 c	78	73	5	7	6	1	14	791	427
Cacoa powder	1 tbsp	3	2	1	0	1	0	1	0	20
Cocoa powder	1 tbsp	3	1	2	0	1	0	1	1	12
Condensed milk, sweetened	1 tbsp	10	10	0	10	2	1	2	24	61
Cooking spray	1 spray	0	0	0	0	0	0	0	0	2

Baking Ingredients & Sweeteners (cont')	Serving Size	Total Carbs (g)	Net Carbs (g)	Fiber (g)	Sugar (g)	Total Fat (g)	Sat Fat (g)	Protein (g)	Sodium (mg)	Calories
Corn starch	1 tbsp	7	7	0	0	0	0	0	1	31
Corn syrup	1 tbsp	16	16	0	6	0	0	0	13	60
Cornmeal	1 c	94	85	9	1	4	1	10	43	442
Erythritol	1tsp	4	1	3	0	0	0	0	0	0
Evaporated milk	1 fl oz	3	3	0	0	2	1	2	33	42
Flaxseed, ground	2 tbsp	4	1	3	0	6	1	3	5	70
Flour, all purpose white	1/4 c	23	22	1	0	0	0	4	0	110
Flour, Almond	1/4 c	4	1	3	1	12	1	5	0	140
Flour, Coconut	2 tbsp	9	3	6	1	2.5	2	3	30	70
Flour, wheat	1/4 c	21	17	4	0	1	0	4	0	100
Honey, raw	1 tbsp	17	17	0	16	0	0	0	1	60
Molasses, dark or light	1 tbsp	16	16	0	12	0	0	0	8	61
Psyllium Husk Powder	1 tsp	4	0	4	0	0	0	0	0	15
Stevia, drops	4	0	0	0	0	0	0	0	0	0
Stevia, packets, single	1	2	0	2	0	0	0	0	0	0
Sugar, brown, packed	1 c	216	216	0	213	0	0	0	62	836
Sugar, white, granulated, cooking	1 c	200	200	0	200	0	0	0	2	774
Sugar, white, granulated, sweetening	1 tsp	4	4	0	4	0	0	0	0	16
Sugar, white, powdered	1 tbsp	8	8	0	7	0	0	0	0	29
Vanilla extract	1 tsp	1	1	0	1	0	0	0	0	13
Vinegar, apple cider	1 tbsp	0	0	0	0	0	0	0	0	0
Vinegar, rice wine	1 tbsp	0	0	0	0	0	0	0	1	3
Vinegar, white distilled	1 tbsp	0	0	0	0	0	0	0	0	0
Xylitol	1 tsp	4	1	3	0	0	0	0	0	10
Yeast, baking, active dry	1 tsp	2	1	1	0	0	0	2	2	13

Spices & Seasonings	Serving Size	Total Carbs (g)	Net Carbs (g)	Fiber (g)	Sugar (g)	Total Fat (g)	Sat Fat (g)	Protein (g)	Sodium (mg)	Calories
Basil, dried	1 tsp	0	0	0	0	0	0	0	1	2
Cayenne Pepper	1 tsp	1	0	1	0	0	0	0	1	6
Chili Powder	1 tsp	1	0	1	0	0	0	0	77	8
Cinnamon	1 tsp	2	1	1	0	0	0	0	0	6
Cloves, ground	1 tsp	2	1	1	0	0	0	0	6	6
Cumin	1 tsp	1	1	1	0	0	0	0	3	8
Garlic Powder	1 tsp	2	2	0	0	0	0	0	2	11
Garlic, minced	1 tsp	1	0	1	0	0	0	0	0	5
Mustard, dried	1 tsp	0	0	0	0	0	0	1	0	9
Nutmeg	1 tsp	1	0	1	0	0	0	0	0	12
Onion Powder	1 tsp	2	2	0	0	0	0	0	2	8
Oregano, dried	1 tsp	1	1	0	0	0	0	0	0	3
Parsley, dried	1 tsp	0	0	0	0	0	0	0	2	2
Rosemary, dried	1 tsp	1	0	1	0	0	0	0	1	4
Salt, garlic	1 tsp	1	1	0	0	0	0	0	968	4
Salt, iodized	1 tsp	0	0	0	0	0	0	0	2326	0
Salt, onion	1 tsp	1	1	0	1	0	0	0	1587	6
Salt, sea	1 tsp	0	0	0	0	0	0	0	145	0
Thyme, dried	1 tsp	1	1	0	0	0	0	0	1	3

Crackers & Chips	Serving Size	Total Carbs (g)	Net Carbs (g)	Fiber (g)	Sugar (g)	Total Fat (g)	Sat Fat (g)	Protein (g)	Sodium (mg)	Calories
Chips, Doritos, single	1	2	2	0	0	1	0	0	19	13
Chips, potato, single	1	1	1	0	0	1	0	0	10	10
Chips, tortilla, single	1	2	2	0	0	1	0	0	13	15
Crackers, Ritz, single	1	2	2	0	0	1	0	0	21	17
Crackers, saltines, single	1	2	2	0	0	0	0	0	28	13
Melba Toast, single	1	2	2	0	0	0	0	0	18	11
Popcorn, home, air popped	1 c	6	5	1	0	0	0	1	1	31
Popcorn, microwave	1 c	4	3	1	0	3	1	1	69	40

Desserts & Other Baked Goods	Serving Size	Total Carbs (g)	Net Carbs (g)	Fiber (g)	Sugar (g)	Total Fat (g)	Sat Fat (g)	Protein (g)	Sodium (mg)	Calories
Breakfast bars, most, single	1	29	28	1	12	8	6	4	108	200
Brownie, chocolate, single	1	24	23	1	18	11	4	3	11	207
Cake, piece or cupcake, single	1	30	29	1	17	6	1	2	290	174
Cake, cheesecake, single slice	1	37	36	1	29	32	15	7	279	455
Cookies, chocolate chip, single	1	10	10	0	7	4	2	1	71	76
Cookies, oatmeal, single	1	11	11	0	6	2	1	1	38	66
Cookies, oreos, single	1	8	8	0	5	2	1	1	47	54
Cookies, vanilla wafer, single	1	3	3	0	2	1	0	0	13	18
Donut, cake, chocolate frosted, single	1	40	39	1	20	19	9	4	340	350
Donut, glazed, single	1	30	29	1	12	14	6	3	330	260
Ice Cream, most flavors	1/2 c	16	15	1	14	7	5	2	53	137
Jello, flavored, sugar free, single container	1	1	0	1	0	0	0	1	55	7
Muffin, bran, single	1	49	44	5	23	10	2	6	428	290
Pie, chocolate cream, single crust, single slice	1	51	48	3	31	23	11	8	212	437
Pie, fruit, double crust, single slice	1	55	53	2	26	21	7	4	298	418
Pudding, chocolate	1/2 c	30	30	0	22	6	2	3	198	185
Pudding, chocolate, sugar free	1/2 c	17	14	3	0	4	2	0	148	85
Sherbet	1/2 c	23	22	1	18	2	1	1	34	107

Beverages	Serving Size	Total Carbs (g)	Net Carbs (g)	Fiber (g)	Sugar (g)	Total Fat (g)	Sat Fat (g)	Protein (g)	Sodium (mg)	Calories
Beer, light	12 fl oz	6	6	0	0	0	0	1	14	103
Beer, reg	12 fl oz	13	13	0	0	0	0	2	14	153
Coffee, ground, decaf	12 fl oz	2	0	2	0	0	0	0	7	0
Coffee, ground, reg	12 fl oz	2	0	2	0	0	0	0	7	4
Hot Chocolate or Hot Cocoa	1 c	31	29	2	25	3	2	1	236	130
Kombucha Tea, cranberry flavored	8 fl oz	7	7	0	2	0	0	0	10	30

Beverages (cont')	Serving Size	Total Carbs (g)	Net Carbs (g)	Fiber (g)	Sugar (g)	Total Fat (g)	Sat Fat (g)	Protein (g)	Sodium (mg)	Calories
Soda, club	12 fl oz	0	0	0	0	0	0	0	75	0
Soda, dark, diet	12 fl oz	0	0	0	0	0	0	0	40	0
Soda, dark, reg	12 fl oz	39	39	0	39	0	0	0	45	140
Soda, light, diet	12 fl oz	0	0	0	0	0	0	0	35	0
Soda, light, reg	12 fl oz	38	38	0	38	0	0	0	65	140
Spirits (Gin, Rum, Vodka, Whiskey)	1.5 fl oz	0	0	0	0	0	0	0	0	97
Sports drink (gatorade)	20 fl oz	34	34	0	34	0	0	0	270	130
Tea, brewed, unsweetened	1 c	1	1	0	0	0	0	0	7	2
Tea, iced, lemon, unsweetened	12 fl oz	0	0	0	0	0	0	0	5	0
Vegetable Juice Cocktail	1 c	9	8	1	6	1	0	2	627	42
Water, zero, flavored	12 fl oz	4	4	0	0	0	0	0	0	0
Wine, dessert, sweet	5 fl oz	20	20	0	11	0	0	0	13	235
Wine, table, red	5 fl oz	4	4	0	1	0	0	0	6	125
Wine, table, white	5 fl oz	4	4	0	1	0	0	0	7	121

Supplements	Serving Size	Total Carbs (g)	Net Carbs (g)	Fiber (g)	Sugar (g)	Total Fat (g)	Sat Fat (g)	Protein (g)	Sodium (mg)	Calories
Bone Broth, beef	1 c	2	2	0	0	0	0	6	240	30
Bone Broth, chicken	1 c	0	0	0	0	1	0	10	240	50
Oil, MCT	1 tbsp	0	0	0	0	14	13	0	0	116
Powder, Collagen	1 scoop	0	0	0	0	0	0	9	25	35
Powder, MCT Oil	1 scoop	1	0	1	0	7	7	1	0	70
Powder, Pea Protein	1 scoop	9	7	2	2	3	0	24	570	160
Powder, Whey Protein	1 scoop	5	4	1	4	2	1	20	100	120

NUTRITION FACTS

alphabetized

Foods In Alphabetical Order	Serving Size	Total Carbs (g)	Net Carbs (g)	Fiber (g)	Sugar (g)	Total Fat (g)	Sat Fat (g)	Protein (g)	Sodium (mg)	Calories
Alcohol, spirits (Gin, Rum, Vodka, Whiskey)	1.5 fl oz	0	0	0	0	0	0	0	0	97
Alfalfa Sprouts, raw	1 c	1	0	1	0	0	0	1	2	8
Almond Butter, unsalted	1 tbsp	3	1	2	1	9	1	3	1	96
Almond Milk, plain, unsweetened	1 c	1	1	0	0	3	0	1	170	36
Almonds, nuts, raw, unsalted, single	3	1	0	1	0	2	0	0	0	21
American Cheese, single slice	1	1	1	0	0	6	3	3	316	69
Anchovies, canned, pieces	6	0	0	0	0	3	0	4	970	40
Apple Juice or Cider, unsweetened	1 c	28	27	1	24	0	0	0	10	114
Apple, raw, w/o skin, single	1	21	19	2	16	0	0	0	0	77
Apple, raw, w/skin, single	1	25	21	4	19	0	0	1	2	95
Apricots, dried	1 tbsp	5	4	1	4	0	0	0	1	20
Apricots, raw, single	1	4	3	1	3	0	0	1	0	17
Artichokes, fresh, boiled, single	1	14	7	7	1	0	0	4	72	64
Artichokes, raw, single	1	14	1	13	1	0	0	4	120	60
Arugula, raw	1 c	1	0	1	0	0	0	1	5	5
Asparagus, fresh or frozen, boiled	1 c	7	3	4	2	0	0	4	25	40
Asparagus, raw, single spear	1	1	1	0	0	0	0	0	0	3
Avocado, black, single	1	12	3	9	0	21	3	3	11	227
Bacon, single slice	1	0	0	0	0	3	1	3	135	37
Bagel, plain, single	1	52	50	2	7	2	1	10	460	270
Baking powder	1 tbsp	4	4	0	0	0	0	0	1463	7
Baking soda	1 tsp	0	0	0	0	0	0	0	1259	0
Bamboo shoots, raw	1/2 c	4	2	2	2	0	0	2	3	21
Banana, raw, single	1	27	24	3	14	0	0	1	1	105
Barley, pearled, cooked	1 c	43	34	9	1	1	0	5	83	193
Basil, dried	1 tsp	0	0	0	0	0	0	0	1	2
Bass, 3 oz fillet	1	0	0	0	0	3	1	15	56	91
BBQ sauce, homemade	1 tbsp	4	4	0	3	0	0	0	99	15
Bean sprouts, mung, raw	1 c	6	4	2	2	0	0	3	6	31

Foods In Alphabetical Order (cont')	Serving Size	Total Carbs (g)	Net Carbs (g)	Fiber (g)	Sugar (g)	Total Fat (g)	Sat Fat (g)	Protein (g)	Sodium (mg)	Calories
Beer, light	12 fl oz	6	6	0	0	0	0	1	14	103
Beer, reg	12 fl oz	13	13	0	0	0	0	2	14	153
Beets, fresh, boiled	1 c	16	13	3	13	0	0	3	121	69
Beets, raw, single	1	8	6	2	6	0	0	1	64	35
Biscuit, homemade, single	1	16	15	1	1	8	2	2	164	149
Bison, steak, 3 oz	1	0	0	0	0	11	5	54	103	332
Black Beans, canned, drained	1 c	45	27	18	1	1	0	14	662	241
Black Beans, dry, cooked	1 c	41	26	15	1	1	0	15	2	227
Black Pepper, ground	1 tsp	2	1	1	0	0	0	0	1	6
Blackberries, frozen	1 c	24	16	8	16	1	0	2	2	97
Blackberries, raw, single	1	1	1	0	0	0	0	0	0	2
Blue Cheese Dressing	1 tbsp	1	1	0	1	8	1	0	98	74
Blue Cheese, crumbled	1 tbsp	0	0	0	0	2	2	2	97	30
Blueberries, frozen	1 c	28	22	6	19	2	0	1	2	117
Blueberries, raw, single	1	0	0	0	0	0	0	0	0	1
Bok Choy, shredded	1 c	2	1	1	1	0	0	1	46	9
Bologna, single slice	1	2	2	0	0	8	3	3	299	95
Bone Broth, beef	1 c	2	2	0	0	0	0	6	240	30
Bone Broth, chicken	1 c	0	0	0	0	1	0	10	240	50
Bratwurst, sausage, single link	1	2	2	0	2	28	8	8	698	230
Brazil Nuts, raw, unsalted, single	3	2	1	1	0	10	2	2	0	93
Bread crumbs, plain	1 c	78	73	5	7	6	1	14	791	427
Bread, wheat, single slice	2	38	32	6	6	3	0	8	300	200
Bread, white, gluten free, single slice	2	18	14	4	4	2	0	2	210	170
Bread, white, single slice	2	29	27	2	5	2	0	4	180	140
Bread, zero carb, single slice	1	7	0	7	0	2	1	7	90	45
Breakfast bars, most, single	1	29	28	1	12	8	6	4	108	200
Brick Cheese, single cracker slice	1	0	0	0	0	3	2	2	50	33
Brie Cheese	1 tbsp	0	0	0	0	4	3	3	94	50

Foods In Alphabetical Order (cont')	Serving Size	Total Carbs (g)	Net Carbs (g)	Fiber (g)	Sugar (g)	Total Fat (g)	Sat Fat (g)	Protein (g)	Sodium (mg)	Calories
Broccoli, fresh, boiled, chopped	1 c	11	6	5	2	1	0	4	64	55
Broccoli, raw, chopped	1 c	6	4	2	2	0	0	3	30	31
Broccoli, raw, single flower	1	1	1	0	0	0	0	0	4	4
Brownie, chocolate, single	1	24	23	1	18	11	4	3	11	207
Brussel Sprouts, fresh, boiled, whole	1 c	11	7	4	3	1	0	4	33	56
Brussel Sprouts, raw, pieces	1 tbsp	1	1	0	0	0	0	0	1	2
Butter, cashew, unsalted	1 tbsp	4	4	0	1	8	2	3	2	94
Butter, ghee	1 tbsp	0	0	0	0	8	8	0	0	112
Butter, margarine	1 tbsp	0	0	0	0	11	2	0	93	99
Butter, peanut, organic, no stir	1 tbsp	2	0	2	1	9	1	3	33	100
Butter, raw, salted	1 tbsp	0	0	0	0	12	7	0	0	102
Butter, sunflower seed	1 tbsp	4	3	1	2	9	1	3	1	99
Butter, tahini, sesame seed butter	1 tbsp	3	2	1	0	8	1	3	17	89
Buttermilk, whole	1 c	12	12	0	12	8	5	8	257	152
Cabbage, green, fresh, cooked	1 c	8	5	3	4	0	0	2	12	35
Cabbage, green, raw, chopped	1 c	5	3	2	3	0	0	1	16	22
Cabbage, red, fresh, cooked	1 c	10	6	4	5	0	0	2	42	44
Cabbage, red, raw, chopped	1 c	7	5	2	3	0	0	1	24	28
Cacoa powder	1 tbsp	3	2	1	0	1	0	1	0	20
Caesar Dressing	1 tbsp	1	1	0	0	9	1	0	178	77
Cake, piece or cupcake, single	1	30	29	1	17	6	1	2	290	174
Calamari, squid, breaded	1 c	18	17	1	1	16	3	23	518	315
Canola Oil	1 tbsp	0	0	0	0	14	1	0	0	120
Cantaloupe, melon, cubed	1 c	13	12	1	13	0	0	1	26	54
Carrots, baby, raw, single	1	1	1	0	1	0	0	0	8	4
Carrots, fresh, cooked, diced	1 c	12	8	4	5	0	0	1	84	51
Carrots, fresh, single	1	6	4	2	3	0	0	1	42	25
Cashew Milk, plain, unsweetened	1 c	1	1	0	0	2	0	1	160	25
Cashews, nuts, raw, unsalted, single	3	2	2	0	0	2	0	1	0	27
Catfish, 6 oz fillet	1	0	0	0	0	10	2	26	170	206

Foods In Alphabetical Order (cont')	Serving Size	Total Carbs (g)	Net Carbs (g)	Fiber (g)	Sugar (g)	Total Fat (g)	Sat Fat (g)	Protein (g)	Sodium (mg)	Calories
Cauliflower, fresh, boiled	1 c	5	2	3	3	0	0	2	19	29
Cauliflower, raw, single flower	1	1	1	0	0	0	0	0	4	3
Caviar	1 tsp	0	0	0	0	1	0	1	80	14
Cayenne Pepper	1 tsp	1	0	1	0	0	0	0	1	6
Celery, fresh, cooked	1 c	6	4	2	4	0	0	1	137	27
Celery, raw, single stalk	1	1	0	1	1	0	0	0	32	6
Cheddar Cheese, shredded	1 c	4	4	0	1	38	21	26	738	457
Cheddar Cheese, single cracker slice	1	0	0	0	0	3	2	2	59	36
Cheesecake, single slice	1	37	36	1	29	32	15	7	279	455
Cherries, frozen	1 c	22	19	3	18	0	0	2	0	88
Cherries, sweet, pitted, single	1	1	1	0	1	0	0	0	0	5
Chia Seeds	1 tbsp	4	1	3	0	3	0	2	2	49
Chicken, breast, baked or roasted, 1/2 breast	1	0	0	0	0	8	2	29	70	193
Chicken, canned, 5 oz	1	2	2	0	0	2	1	23	500	127
Chicken, cornish game hen, roasted, 3 oz	1	0	0	0	0	16	4	19	54	220
Chicken, leg, breaded and fried	1	3	3	0	0	16	4	30	99	285
Chicken, whole, roasted, 3 oz	1	0	0	0	0	12	3	23	530	210
Chili Powder	1 tsp	1	0	1	0	0	0	0	77	8
Chocolate Chip Cookies, single	1	10	10	0	7	4	2	1	71	76
Chocolate Milk, whole	1 c	26	24	2	24	9	5	8	150	208
Cilantro, raw, single sprig	1	0	0	0	0	0	0	0	1	1
Cinnamon	1 tsp	2	1	1	0	0	0	0	0	6
Clams, fresh, cooked, single	1	0	0	0	0	0	0	3	14	18
Clementine, single	1	9	8	1	7	0	0	1	1	35
Cloves, ground	1 tsp	2	1	1	0	0	0	0	6	6
Cocoa powder	1 tbsp	3	1	2	0	1	0	1	1	12
Coconut Milk, canned, unsweetened	1 fl oz	1	1	0	1	4	4	0	10	46
Coconut Oil	1 tbsp	0	0	0	0	14	11	0	0	122
Coconut Water	1 fl oz	1	1	0	1	0	0	0	0	6
Coconut, whole, single	1	61	25	36	25	133	118	13	80	1405

Foods In Alphabetical Order (cont')	Serving Size	Total Carbs (g)	Net Carbs (g)	Fiber (g)	Sugar (g)	Total Fat (g)	Sat Fat (g)	Protein (g)	Sodium (mg)	Calories
Cod, 4 oz fillet	1	0	0	0	0	0	0	18	121	76
Coffee Cream, powdered	1 tsp	1	1	0	0	1	0	0	2	10
Coffee, ground, decaf	12 fl oz	2	0	2	0	0	0	0	7	0
Coffee, ground, reg	12 fl oz	2	0	2	0	0	0	0	7	4
Colby Cheese, single slice	1	1	1	0	0	9	6	7	169	110
Coleslaw	1 c	12	9	3	8	37	6	2	344	384
Collagen Powder	1 scoop	0	0	0	0	0	0	9	25	35
Collards, fresh, cooked	1 c	11	8	3	1	1	0	5	29	63
Condensed milk, sweetened	1 tbsp	10	10	0	10	2	1	2	24	61
Cooking spray	1 spray	0	0	0	0	0	0	0	0	2
Corn Oil	1 tbsp	0	0	0	0	14	2	0	0	123
Corn starch	1 tbsp	7	7	0	0	0	0	0	1	31
Corn syrup	1 tbsp	16	16	0	6	0	0	0	13	60
Corn, canned, cream	1 c	46	43	3	8	1	0	5	668	184
Corn, canned, whole	1 c	24	21	3	7	2	0	4	336	110
Corn, frozen, whole kernel	1 c	32	28	4	5	1	0	4	2	134
Corn, single ear, cooked	1	22	19	3	5	2	0	4	1	99
Corn, single ear, raw	1	17	15	2	3	1	0	3	14	77
Corned Beef, single slice	1	0	0	0	0	1	1	4	281	30
Cornmeal	1 c	94	85	9	1	4	1	10	43	442
Cottage Cheese, 2%	1 c	11	11	0	9	5	3	24	696	183
Cottage Cheese, whole	1 c	7	7	0	6	9	4	23	764	206
Crab leg, single	1	0	0	0	0	0	0	8	168	35
Crab meat	3 oz	0	0	0	0	1	0	19	320	90
Cranberries, dried, sweetened	1 tbsp	24	22	2	21	0	0	0	1	87
Cranberry Juice, unsweetened	1 fl oz	4	4	0	3	0	0	0	1	13
Crayfish or crawfish	1 c	0	0	0	0	3	0	41	231	201
Cream Cheese	1 c	7	7	0	6	9	4	23	764	206
Croissant Roll, single	1	27	26	1	4	15	9	5	75	260
Croutons, seasoned, 1 svg of 7g	1	4	3	1	0	1	0	1	76	33

35

Foods In Alphabetical Order (cont')	Serving Size	Total Carbs (g)	Net Carbs (g)	Fiber (g)	Sugar (g)	Total Fat (g)	Sat Fat (g)	Protein (g)	Sodium (mg)	Calories
Cucumber, raw, single slice	1	0	0	0	0	0	0	0	0	1
Cumin	1 tsp	1	1	1	0	0	0	0	3	8
Dates, pitted, medjool, single	1	18	16	2	16	0	0	0	0	67
Deli Meat, turkey, single slice	1	0	0	0	0	0	0	4	206	21
Dinner Roll, sweet, single	1	16	15	1	5	2	1	3	76	96
Dinner Roll, wheat, single	1	13	12	1	1	2	1	2	147	76
Donut, cake, chocolate frosted, single	1	40	39	1	20	19	9	4	340	350
Donut, glazed, single	1	30	29	1	12	14	6	3	330	260
Doritos, chips, single	1	2	2	0	0	1	0	0	19	13
Edam Cheese, single cracker slice	1	0	0	0	0	7	5	7	270	89
Edamame, fresh, cooked	1 c	20	12	8	3	12	1	22	25	254
Egg, substitute, white, single	1	0	0	0	0	0	0	5	171	24
Egg, white, cooked, single	1	0	0	0	0	0	0	4	55	17
Egg, whole, raw or cooked, single	1	1	1	0	1	5	2	6	62	78
Egg, yolk, cooked, single	1	1	1	0	0	4	2	3	8	54
Eggplant, fresh, cooked	1 c	9	6	3	3	0	0	1	1	35
Eggplant, raw, peeled, single	1	27	13	14	16	1	0	5	9	115
English Muffin, wheat, single whole	1	27	23	4	5	1	0	6	240	134
English Muffin, white, single whole	1	25	23	2	2	1	0	5	242	129
Erythritol	1tsp	4	1	3	0	0	0	0	0	0
Evaporated milk	1 fl oz	3	3	0	0	2	1	2	33	42
Fennel, raw, sliced	1 c	6	3	3	3	0	0	1	45	27
Feta Cheese, crumbled	1 tbsp	0	0	0	0	2	1	1	86	25
Figs, dried, single	1	5	4	1	4	0	0	0	1	21
Figs, raw, single	1	8	7	1	7	0	0	0	0	30
Fish sticks, single stick	1	3	3	0	1	2	0	2	52	36
Flank, steak, 3 oz	1	0	0	0	0	7	3	24	48	165
Flaxseed Oil	1 tbsp	0	0	0	0	14	1	0	0	120
Flaxseed, ground	2 tbsp	4	1	3	0	6	1	3	5	70
Flaxseeds, raw	1 tbsp	2	0	2	0	3	0	1	2	37

Foods In Alphabetical Order (cont')	Serving Size	Total Carbs (g)	Net Carbs (g)	Fiber (g)	Sugar (g)	Total Fat (g)	Sat Fat (g)	Protein (g)	Sodium (mg)	Calories
Flour, all purpose white	1/4 c	23	22	1	0	0	0	4	0	110
Flour, almond	1/4 c	4	1	3	1	12	1	5	0	140
Flour, coconut	2 tbsp	9	3	6	1	2.5	2	3	30	70
Flour, wheat	1/4 c	21	17	4	0	1	0	4	0	100
French Fries, potatoes, baked, steak, single	1	2	2	0	0	1	0	0	29	14
French Fries, potatoes, fried, single	1 c	43	39	4	2	15	2	4	218	319
French Toast, white, homemade, single	1	15	14	1	3	5	1	5	184	125
Garbanzo Beans (chick peas), canned, drained	1 c	37	26	11	7	5	0	12	403	228
Garbanzo Beans (chick peas), dry, cooked	1 c	45	32	13	8	4	0	15	12	269
Garlic Powder	1 tsp	2	2	0	0	0	0	0	2	11
Garlic, minced	1 tsp	1	0	1	0	0	0	0	0	5
Garlic, raw, single clove	1	1	1	0	0	0	0	0	1	5
Gin	1.5 fl oz	0	0	0	0	0	0	0	0	97
Goat Cheese, soft, crumbled	1 tbsp	0	0	0	0	2	1	2	40	23
Goat Milk	1 c	11	11	0	11	10	7	9	122	169
Gouda Cheese, single cracker slice	1	0	0	0	0	3	2	2	74	32
Grape, juice, unsweetened	1 fl oz	5	5	0	5	0	0	0	2	19
Grapefruit, juice	1 fl oz	3	3	0	2	0	0	0	0	12
Grapefruit, raw, single	1	27	23	4	18	0	0	2	0	108
Grapes, raw, seedless, single	1	1	1	0	1	0	0	0	0	3
Green Beans, snap, fresh, cooked	1 c	10	6	4	5	0	0	2	1	44
Green Beans, snap, raw, single	1	0	0	0	0	0	0	0	0	2
Green Onions, (scallions), tops and bulb, raw, s	1	1	1	0	1	0	0	0	2	5
Ground beef, 85% lean	1 c	0	0	0	0	31	12	56	139	520
Gruyere Cheese, single cracker slice	1	0	0	0	0	3	2	3	64	37
Guacamole	1 tbsp	1	0	1	0	1	0	0	59	14
Haddock, 7 oz fillet	1	0	0	0	0	1	0	30	392	135
Half and Half, cream	1 tbsp	1	1	0	1	2	1	1	9	19
Halibut, 14 oz	1	0	0	0	0	5	1	72	261	353
Ham, honey roasted, 2 oz	1	4	4	0	4	3	1	10	540	80

Foods In Alphabetical Order (cont')	Serving Size	Total Carbs (g)	Net Carbs (g)	Fiber (g)	Sugar (g)	Total Fat (g)	Sat Fat (g)	Protein (g)	Sodium (mg)	Calories
Hamburger/Hot Dog Bun, wheat, single	1	18	15	3	2	2	0	5	196	108
Hamburger/Hot Dog Bun, white, single	1	22	21	1	3	2	0	4	212	120
Hashbrowns, potatoes	1 c	15	13	2	1	0	0	2	25	70
Hazelnuts, nuts, single	3	1	1	0	0	3	0	1	0	26
Herring, 7 oz fillet	1	0	0	0	0	26	6	30	137	360
Honey, raw	1 tbsp	17	17	0	16	0	0	0	1	60
Horseradish	1 tbsp	2	1	1	1	0	0	0	63	7
Hot Chocolate or Hot Cocoa	1 c	31	29	2	25	3	2	1	236	130
Hot Pepper Sauce	1 tsp	0	0	0	0	0	0	0	124	1
Hummus	1 tbsp	3	2	1	1	1	0	1	66	27
Ice Cream, most flavors	1/2 c	16	15	1	14	7	5	2	53	137
Italian Dressing	1 tbsp	2	2	0	2	3	0	0	146	35
Italian Sausage, single link	1	3	3	0	1	21	7	14	557	258
Jalapeno Peppers, canned	1 oz	2	2	0	1	0	0	1	25	10
Jalapeno Peppers, raw, single	1	1	1	0	1	0	0	0	0	4
Jello, flavored, sugar free, single container	1	1	0	1	0	0	0	1	55	7
Jelly, grape, squeezable	1 tbsp	13	13	0	12	0	0	0	5	50
Jicama, cooked	1 c	12	5	7	2	0	0	1	5	51
Jicama, raw, sliced	1 c	3	1	2	1	0	0	0	2	14
Kale, fresh, cooked	1 c	7	4	3	2	0	0	3	30	36
Kale, raw	1 c	1	0	1	0	0	0	1	6	8
Kefir, lowfat, flavored	8 fl oz	20	20	0	20	2	2	11	125	139
Kefir, whole, plain	8 fl oz	11	11	0	10	8	5	12	130	160
Ketchup (Catsup)	1 tbsp	4	4	0	3	0	0	0	136	15
Kidney Beans, canned, drained	1 c	38	28	10	7	2	0	14	409	220
Kidney Beans, dry, cooked	1 c	40	29	11	1	1	0	15	2	225
Kiwi, raw, single	1	10	8	2	6	0	0	1	2	42
Kombucha Tea, cranberry flavored	8 fl oz	7	7	0	2	0	0	0	10	30
Lard (made from animal fats)	1 tbsp	0	0	0	0	13	5	0	0	116

Foods In Alphabetical Order (cont')	Serving Size	Total Carbs (g)	Net Carbs (g)	Fiber (g)	Sugar (g)	Total Fat (g)	Sat Fat (g)	Protein (g)	Sodium (mg)	Calories
Leeks, fresh, cooked, single	1	9	8	1	3	0	0	1	12	38
Leeks, raw, single	1	13	11	2	4	0	0	1	18	54
Lemon, juice	1 tbsp	1	1	0	0	0	0	0	0	3
Lemon, raw, single	1	4	3	1	1	0	0	0	1	12
Lentil Beans, canned, drained	1 c	40	28	12	1	1	0	18	471	230
Lentil Beans, dry, cooked	1 c	40	28	12	1	1	0	18	4	230
Lettuce, Boston, Bib, Butterhead	1 c	1	0	1	1	0	0	1	3	7
Lettuce, Iceberg	1 c	2	1	1	1	0	0	1	6	8
Lettuce, Romaine	1 c	2	1	1	1	0	0	1	4	8
Lime, raw, single	1	7	5	2	1	0	0	1	1	20
Liverwurst, sausage, single slice	1	0	0	0	0	5	2	3	155	59
Lobster, 1 lb	1	0	0	0	0	1	0	22	574	105
Macadamia Nuts, single	3	1	0	1	0	6	1	1	0	56
Mackerel, 8 oz fillet	1	0	0	0	0	18	5	45	194	354
Mango, raw, single	1	50	45	5	46	1	0	3	3	202
Mashed Potatoes	1 c	44	40	4	3	9	2	4	359	268
Mayonnaise	1 tbsp	0	0	0	0	10	2	0	87	94
MCT Oil	1 tbsp	0	0	0	0	14	13	0	0	116
MCT Oil, powder	1 scoop	1	0	1	0	7	7	1	0	70
Melba Toast, single	1	2	2	0	0	0	0	0	18	11
Melon, honeydew, cubed	1 c	17	15	2	16	0	0	1	34	69
Milk, cow, 2%	1 c	12	12	0	12	5	3	8	115	122
Milk, cow, whole	1 c	12	12	0	12	8	5	8	105	149
Miso	1 tbsp	4	3	1	1	1	0	2	641	34
Mixed nuts, dry, roasted, salted, single	3	1	1	0	0	2	0	1	15	26
Molasses, dark or light	1 tbsp	16	16	0	12	0	0	0	8	61
Mozzarella Cheese, part skim, shredded	1 c	6	6	0	2	22	13	27	753	333
Muffin, bran, single	1	49	44	5	23	10	2	6	428	290
Mushrooms, canned	1 c	8	4	4	4	1	0	3	663	39
Mushrooms, fresh, cooked	1 c	8	5	3	4	1	0	3	3	44

Foods In Alphabetical Order (cont')	Serving Size	Total Carbs (g)	Net Carbs (g)	Fiber (g)	Sugar (g)	Total Fat (g)	Sat Fat (g)	Protein (g)	Sodium (mg)	Calories
Mushrooms, raw, single	1	1	1	0	0	0	0	1	1	4
Mustard Greens, fresh, cooked	1 c	6	3	3	2	1	0	4	13	36
Mustard, dried	1 tsp	0	0	0	0	0	0	1	0	9
Mustard, sauce	1 tbsp	1	0	1	0	1	0	1	172	9
Navy Beans, canned, drained	1 c	47	28	19	1	1	0	15	701	255
Navy Beans, dry, cooked	1 c	47	28	19	1	1	0	15	0	255
Nectarine, raw, single	1	15	13	2	11	1	0	2	0	63
Nutella	1 tbsp	12	11	1	10	6	1	1	8	100
Nutmeg	1 tsp	1	0	1	0	0	0	0	0	12
Oatmeal Cookies, single	1	11	11	0	6	2	1	1	38	66
Oatmeal, cooked	1 c	55	47	8	1	5	1	11	5	307
Okra, fresh, cooked	1 c	7	3	4	3	0	0	3	10	35
Olive Oil, extra virgin, cold pressed	1 tbsp	0	0	0	0	14	2	0	0	119
Olives, black, raw, single	1	0	0	0	0	0	0	0	29	5
Olives, green, raw, single	1	0	0	0	0	1	0	0	53	5
Onion Dip	1 tbsp	2	2	0	1	2	2	1	105	30
Onion Powder	1 tsp	2	2	0	0	0	0	0	2	8
Onions, white, yellow, red, fresh, cooked	1 c	13	11	2	6	0	0	2	4	56
Onions, white, yellow, red, raw, single	1	10	8	2	5	0	0	1	4	44
Orange Juice	1 fl oz	3	3	0	3	0	0	0	0	14
Orange, raw, single	1	15	12	3	12	0	0	1	0	62
Oregano, dried	1 tsp	1	1	0	0	0	0	0	0	3
Oreos, cookies, single	1	8	8	0	5	2	1	1	47	54
Oysters, canned, 8 oz	1	1	1	0	0	5	1	15	234	142
Oysters, fresh, cooked	1 c	2	2	0	0	11	3	46	520	400
Pancake, homemade, single	1	13	13	0	3	4	1	3	306	99
Papaya, raw, single	1	33	28	5	24	1	0	1	24	131
Parmesan Cheese, fresh or dry, grated	1 tbsp	1	1	0	0	2	1	2	102	27
Parsley, dried	1 tsp	0	0	0	0	0	0	0	2	2
Parsley, raw	1 tbsp	0	0	0	0	0	0	0	2	1

Foods In Alphabetical Order (cont')	Serving Size	Total Carbs (g)	Net Carbs (g)	Fiber (g)	Sugar (g)	Total Fat (g)	Sat Fat (g)	Protein (g)	Sodium (mg)	Calories
Parsnip, cooked, single	1	17	4	3	5	0	0	1	10	70
Pasta Noodles, cooked	1 c	43	40	3	1	1	0	8	1	221
Pastrami, beef, single slice	1	0	0	0	0	2	1	6	379	41
Pea Protein, powder	1 scoop	9	7	2	2	3	0	24	570	160
Peach, raw, single	1	14	12	2	13	0	0	1	0	59
Peanut Oil	1 tbsp	0	0	0	0	14	2	0	0	120
Peanuts, nuts, single	3	0	0	0	0	1	0	1	1	15
Pear, raw, single	1	27	21	6	17	0	0	1	0	102
Peas, green, canned	1 c	20	11	9	5	1	0	8	478	119
Peas, green, fresh or frozen, cooked	1 c	23	16	7	7	0	0	8	115	125
Peas, snowpeas, raw, single pod	1	0	0	0	0	0	0	0	0	1
Pecans, nuts, single	3	1	0	1	0	6	1	1	0	62
Perch, 2 oz fillet	1	0	0	0	0	1	0	9	174	48
Pesto, homemade	1 tbsp	1	1	0	0	8	2	1	57	79
Pickle, single slice	1	0	0	0	0	0	0	0	169	2
Pickle, sour, single whole	1	2	1	1	1	0	0	0	785	8
Pie, chocolate cream, single crust, single slice	1	51	48	3	31	23	11	8	212	437
Pie, fruit, double crust, single slice	1	55	53	2	26	21	7	4	298	418
Pike, 14 oz fillet	1	0	0	0	0	3	1	77	152	350
Pine Nuts	1 tbsp	2	1	1	1	5	1	1	6	53
Pineapple Juice	1 fl oz	4	4	0	3	0	0	0	1	17
Pineapple, raw, chunks	1 c	22	20	2	16	0	0	1	2	83
Pinto Beans, canned, drained	1 c	35	25	10	1	2	0	12	409	195
Pinto Beans, dry, cooked	1 c	45	30	15	1	1	0	15	2	245
Pistachios, nuts, single	3	1	1	0	0	1	0	0	0	10
Pita, white, single	1	33	32	1	0	1	0	6	322	165
Pita, whole grain, single	1	32	28	4	2	1	0	6	300	149
Plantain, raw, single	1	57	53	4	27	1	0	2	7	218
Plum, raw, single	1	6	5	1	6	0	0	0	0	25
Polish Kielbasa, sausage, single link	1	2	2	0	2	20	7	8	670	221

Foods In Alphabetical Order (cont')	Serving Size	Total Carbs (g)	Net Carbs (g)	Fiber (g)	Sugar (g)	Total Fat (g)	Sat Fat (g)	Protein (g)	Sodium (mg)	Calories
Pomegranate, raw, single	1	53	42	11	39	3	0	5	9	234
Popcorn, home, air popped	1 c	6	5	1	0	0	0	1	1	31
Popcorn, microwave	1 c	4	3	1	0	3	1	1	69	40
Pork, chops, single	1	0	0	0	0	7	2	46	105	256
Pork, ground	1 c	0	0	0	0	46	16	59	193	652
Pork, loin, 3 oz	1	0	0	0	0	3	1	22	49	122
Pork, ribs, spare, single	1	0	0	0	0	11	4	10	33	139
Potato Chips, single	1	1	1	0	0	1	0	0	10	10
Potato Salad, homemade	1 c	28	25	3	0	21	4	7	1323	358
Potato, baked, skin not eaten, single	1	28	26	2	2	0	0	3	7	122
Potato, boiled w/o skin, single	1	33	30	3	2	0	0	3	8	144
Prune Juice, unsweetened	1 fl oz	6	6	0	5	0	0	0	1	23
Prunes, dried	1 tbsp	7	6	1	4	0	0	0	0	26
Psyllium Husk Powder	1 tsp	4	0	4	0	0	0	0	0	15
Pudding, chocolate	1/2 c	30	30	0	22	6	2	3	198	185
Pudding, chocolate, sugar free	1/2 c	17	14	3	0	4	2	2	148	85
Pumpkin Seeds, raw, unsalted	1/4 c	4	2	2	0	13	3	11	0	180
Quinoa, cooked	1 c	39	34	5	2	4	0	8	13	222
Radish, raw, single	1	0	0	0	0	0	0	0	2	1
Raisins, uncooked	1 tbsp	7	7	0	5	0	0	0	1	27
Ranch Dressing, creamy	1 tbsp	0	0	0	0	7	1	0	210	61
Raspberries, raw, single	1	0	0	0	0	0	0	0	0	1
Relish, sweet pickle	1 tsp	2	2	0	2	0	0	0	41	7
Rhubarb, cooked, unsweetened	1 c	5	2	3	2	0	0	2	2	17
Rhubarb, raw, stalk	1	2	1	1	1	0	0	1	2	11
Rib roast, 3 oz	1	0	0	0	0	20	9	20	43	258
Ribeye, 4 oz	1	0	0	0	0	12	6	21	60	190
Rice Milk, plain, unsweetened	1 c	7	4	3	2	3	0	0	135	52
Rice, brown, cooked	1 c	52	49	3	1	2	1	6	8	249
Rice, white, cooked	1 c	45	44	1	0	0	0	4	2	205

Foods In Alphabetical Order (cont')	Serving Size	Total Carbs (g)	Net Carbs (g)	Fiber (g)	Sugar (g)	Total Fat (g)	Sat Fat (g)	Protein (g)	Sodium (mg)	Calories
Ricotta Cheese, part skim	1 c	13	13	0	1	20	12	28	243	340
Ricotta Cheese, whole	1 c	8	8	0	5	32	20	28	207	428
Ritz Crackers, single	1	2	2	0	0	1	0	0	21	17
Romano Cheese, fresh or dry, grated	1 tbsp	1	1	0	0	2	1	2	113	26
Rosemary, dried	1 tsp	1	0	1	0	0	0	0	1	4
Round roast, 3 oz	1	0	0	0	0	9	3	24	32	180
Rum	1.5 fl oz	0	0	0	0	0	0	0	0	97
Rump roast, 4 oz	1	0	0	0	0	14	5	23	60	220
Safflower Oil	1 tbsp	0	0	0	0	14	1	0	0	120
Salami, pork and beef, single slice	1	0	0	0	0	5	2	4	209	57
Salmon, wild alaskan, canned	1/4 c	0	0	0	0	7	2	13	230	110
Salmon, wild alaskan, fresh	6 oz	0	0	0	0	10	2	36	190	230
Salsa	1 tbsp	1	1	0	1	0	0	0	115	5
Salt, garlic	1 tsp	1	1	0	0	0	0	0	968	4
Salt, iodized	1 tsp	0	0	0	0	0	0	0	2326	0
Salt, onion	1 tsp	1	1	0	1	0	0	0	1587	6
Salt, sea	1 tsp	0	0	0	0	0	0	0	145	0
Saltines, crackers, single	1	2	2	0	0	0	0	0	28	13
Sardines, canned, water, 4 oz	1	0	0	0	0	9	3	21	118	164
Sauerkraut	1 c	10	3	7	3	0	0	2	1560	45
Sausage, breakfast, single patty	1	0	0	0	0	15	5	5	347	153
Scallops	1 c	13	13	0	0	2	1	50	1637	272
Seaweed, dulse, dried	1 oz	7	6	1	0	1	0	10	85	62
Sesame Oil	1 tbsp	0	0	0	0	14	2	0	0	120
Sherbet	1/2 c	23	22	1	18	2	1	1	34	107
Short ribs, 3 oz	1	0	0	0	0	13	4	25	64	213
Shrimp, breaded	1 c	31	30	1	3	17	3	15	737	335
Shrimp, frozen	1 c	2	2	0	0	3	1	33	1373	173
Sirloin, 3 oz	1	0	0	0	0	8	3	25	52	180
Smelt	1 c	0	0	0	0	8	1	56	189	304

Foods In Alphabetical Order (cont')	Serving Size	Total Carbs (g)	Net Carbs (g)	Fiber (g)	Sugar (g)	Total Fat (g)	Sat Fat (g)	Protein (g)	Sodium (mg)	Calories
Snapper, 8 oz fillet	1	0	0	0	0	3	1	45	97	218
Soda, club	12 fl oz	0	0	0	0	0	0	0	75	0
Soda, dark, diet	12 fl oz	0	0	0	0	0	0	0	40	0
Soda, dark, reg	12 fl oz	39	39	0	39	0	0	0	45	140
Soda, light, diet	12 fl oz	0	0	0	0	0	0	0	35	0
Soda, light, reg	12 fl oz	38	38	0	38	0	0	0	65	140
Sour Cream	1 tbsp	1	1	0	1	3	2	0	4	29
Soy Milk, plain, unsweetened	1 c	4	1	3	1	4	1	8	85	74
Soy Sauce	1 tbsp	1	1	0	0	0	0	1	875	8
Spaghetti Sauce, homemade	1 c	15	10	5	9	10	2	3	927	146
Spinach, canned	1 c	7	2	5	1	1	0	6	420	49
Spinach, frozen, cooked	1 c	9	2	7	1	2	0	8	184	65
Spinach, raw	1 c	1	0	1	0	0	0	1	24	7
Spirulina, seaweed, raw	1 oz	1	1	0	0	0	0	2	28	7
Sports drink (gatorade)	20 fl oz	34	34	0	34	0	0	0	270	130
Squash, butternut, baked	1 c	22	15	7	4	0	0	2	8	82
Squash, spaghetti, baked	1 c	10	8	2	4	0	0	1	28	42
Stevia, drops	4	0	0	0	0	0	0	0	0	0
Stevia, packets, single	1	2	0	2	0	0	0	0	0	0
Stew beef, cubed	1 c	0	0	0	0	20	8	36	77	335
Strawberries, frozen, unsweetened	1 c	20	15	5	10	0	0	1	4	77
Strawberries, raw, single	1	1	1	0	1	0	0	0	0	4
Sugar, brown, packed	1 c	216	216	0	213	0	0	0	62	836
Sugar, white, granulated, cooking	1 c	200	200	0	200	0	0	0	2	774
Sugar, white, granulated, sweetening	1 tsp	4	4	0	4	0	0	0	0	16
Sugar, white, powdered	1 tbsp	8	8	0	7	0	0	0	0	29
Summer Sausage, beef, single slice	1	0	0	0	0	6	3	3	328	71
Sunflower Oil	1 tbsp	0	0	0	0	14	1	0	0	120
Sunflower Seeds	1/4 c	7	4	3	1	18	2	7	3	204

Foods In Alphabetical Order (cont')	Serving Size	Total Carbs (g)	Net Carbs (g)	Fiber (g)	Sugar (g)	Total Fat (g)	Sat Fat (g)	Protein (g)	Sodium (mg)	Calories
Sweet Peppers, fresh, cooked, chopped	1 c	9	8	1	7	0	0	1	3	38
Sweet Peppers, raw, single	1	7	4	3	5	0	0	1	5	37
Sweet Potato (yam), baked, single	1	24	20	4	7	0	0	2	41	103
Swiss Cheese, single slice	1	0	0	0	0	7	4	6	39	83
Syrup, maple, organic	1 tbsp	13	13	0	13	0	0	0	2	50
Syrup, pancake	1 tbsp	14	14	0	8	0	0	0	12	51
T-bone, 4 oz	1	0	0	0	0	19	8	21	60	260
Tangerine (mandarin), raw, single	1	12	10	2	9	0	0	1	2	47
Tartar Sauce	1 tbsp	1	1	0	0	10	2	0	145	95
Tea, brewed, unsweetened	1 c	1	1	0	0	0	0	0	7	2
Tea, iced, lemon, unsweetened	12 fl oz	0	0	0	0	0	0	0	5	0
Tempeh, single patty	1	17	9	8	6	25	6	46	20	436
Tenderloin, 3 oz	1	0	0	0	0	15	6	23	46	227
Thyme, dried	1 tsp	1	1	0	0	0	0	0	1	3
Tofu, single slice	1	2	2	0	1	2	0	6	30	52
Tomato Sauce	1 c	13	9	4	9	1	0	3	1161	59
Tomato, canned	1 c	8	3	5	6	1	0	2	276	38
Tomato, cherry, single	1	1	1	0	0	0	0	0	1	3
Tomato, fresh, cooked	1 c	10	8	2	6	0	0	2	26	43
Tomato, raw, single	1	5	3	2	3	0	0	1	6	22
Tomato, sundried, jar w/oil	3 pcs	4	2	2	3	1	0	1	220	30
Tortilla Chips, single	1	2	2	0	0	1	0	0	13	15
Tortilla, corn, single	1	11	10	1	0	1	0	1	11	52
Tortilla, flour, single	1	26	25	1	1	3	1	4	400	140
Trout, rainbow, 3 oz fillet	1	0	0	0	0	5	1	17	43	119
Tuna, steaks, 5 oz	1	0	0	0	0	1	0	17	25	75
Tuna, white, canned, 5 oz	1	0	0	0	0	4	1	31	65	165
Turkey, ground	1 c	0	0	0	0	40	11	58	196	596
Turkey, whole, roasted, 3 oz	1	0	0	0	0	6	2	24	88	161

45

Foods In Alphabetical Order (cont')	Serving Size	Total Carbs (g)	Net Carbs (g)	Fiber (g)	Sugar (g)	Total Fat (g)	Sat Fat (g)	Protein (g)	Sodium (mg)	Calories
Turnip, fresh, cooked, single	1	6	4	2	4	0	0	1	19	26
Turnip, raw, single	1	8	6	2	5	0	0	1	82	34
Vanilla extract	1 tsp	1	1	0	1	0	0	0	0	13
Vanilla Wafer, cookies, single	1	3	3	0	2	1	0	0	13	18
Veal, cutlets, 3 oz	1	0	0	0	0	2	1	27	75	128
Veal, ground	1 c	0	0	0	0	13	5	57	197	355
Vegetable Juice Cocktail	1 c	9	8	1	6	1	0	2	627	42
Vegetable Oil	1 tbsp	0	0	0	0	14	2	0	0	120
Venison, stew meat	1 c	0	0	0	0	8	3	74	133	388
Vienna Sausage, single link	1	0	0	0	0	3	1	2	141	38
Vinaigrette Dressing, oil	1 tbsp	0	0	0	0	9	1	0	197	82
Vinegar, apple cidar	1 tbsp	0	0	0	0	0	0	0	0	0
Vinegar, rice wine	1 tbsp	0	0	0	0	0	0	0	1	3
Vinegar, white distilled	1 tbsp	0	0	0	0	0	0	0	0	0
Vodka	1.5 fl oz	0	0	0	0	0	0	0	0	97
Waffle, homemade, single	1	31	30	1	5	17	5	7	461	299
Waffle, plain, frozen, single	1	15	14	1	2	3	1	2	223	100
Walleye, 6 oz fillet	1	0	0	0	0	2	0	30	81	148
Walnut Oil	1 tbsp	0	0	0	0	14	1	0	0	120
Walnuts, nuts, single halves	3	1	1	0	0	4	0	1	0	37
Water, Zero, flavored	12 fl oz	4	4	0	0	0	0	0	0	0
Watercress, raw	1 c	0	0	0	0	0	0	1	14	4
Watermelon, cubed	1 c	12	11	1	9	0	0	1	2	46
Weiner, hot dog, single link	1	1	0	1	1	13	4	7	530	140
Whey Protein powder	1 scoop	5	4	1	4	2	1	20	100	120
Whipping Cream, heavy	1 fl oz	1	1	0	1	11	7	1	8	101
Whiskey	1.5 fl oz	0	0	0	0	0	0	0	0	97
White Beans, canned, drained	1 c	56	43	13	1	1	0	19	891	299
White Beans, dry, cooked	1 c	48	35	13	1	1	0	18	11	263
Whitefish, 7 oz fillet	1	0	0	0	0	12	2	38	100	265

Foods In Alphabetical Order (cont')	Serving Size	Total Carbs (g)	Net Carbs (g)	Fiber (g)	Sugar (g)	Total Fat (g)	Sat Fat (g)	Protein (g)	Sodium (mg)	Calories
Wine, dessert, sweet	5 fl oz	20	20	0	11	0	0	0	13	235
Wine, table, red	5 fl oz	4	4	0	1	0	0	0	6	125
Wine, table, white	5 fl oz	4	4	0	1	0	0	0	7	121
Worcheshire Sauce	1 tsp	1	1	0	1	0	0	0	56	5
Xylitol	1 tsp	4	1	3	0	0	0	0	0	10
Yeast, baking, active dry	1 tsp	2	1	1	0	0	0	2	2	13
Yogurt, greek, nonfat, plain	6 oz	6	6	0	6	1	0	17	61	100
Yogurt, lowfat, flavored	6 oz	34	33	1	27	3	2	5	67	180
Yogurt, lowfat, plain	1 c	17	17	0	17	4	3	13	172	154
Yogurt, plain, whole	1 c	11	11	0	11	8	5	9	113	150
Zucchini, fresh, cooked	1 c	6	4	2	4	1	0	2	6	32
Zucchini, raw, single	1	6	4	2	5	1	0	2	16	33

KETO RECIPES

https://blog.paleohacks.com/paleo-egg-bake/

8 eggs
3 slices bacon
½ cup peppers
¼ cup onions
Pepper to taste

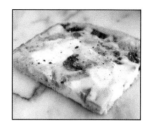

Procedure

Preheat oven to 350°F.
Whisk eggs together in a large bowl and set aside.
Cook 3 slices of bacon over skillet.
While bacon is cooking, chop peppers and onions.
Add peppers and onions to eggs.
Once bacon done, remove from heat, wait 5 minutes or so until cooled a bit and break into tiny pieces, add bacon to eggs.
Grease a baking dish with a bit of coconut oil and pour eggs into dish; set into oven and bake for at least 30 minutes. (Every oven is different, so be sure to keep an eye on your eggs. You may need to leave them in for an additional 5-10 minutes.)
Cut and enjoy!

Servings: 3

https://www.ruled.me/bacon-and-roasted-garlic-guacamole/

2 medium Haas avocados
4 slices bacon
⅓ medium size red bell pepper
¼ small size onion
1 tablespoon roasted garlic
⅓ cup chopped cilantro
½ juice of lime
Salt and pepper to taste

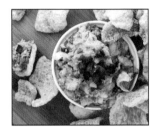

Slice bacon into small cubes using scissors. Add into a hot pan and cook until crisp. Set aside for later.

Slice avocados and take the pit out. Add to a bowl with the crushed roasted garlic.

Slice your vegetables and cilantro, then add to the bowl. Add your bacon (along with the grease) and mix well.

Add lime juice and salt and pepper to taste, then give it one final mix.

Servings: 3

Simple, Delicious Guacamole

https://www.ruled.me/simple-delicious-guacamole/

2 whole Hass avocados
⅓ medium red onion
1 medium jalapeño
2 tablespoons pre-made salsa
1 tablespoon fresh lime juice
Salt and pepper to taste
½ bunch (½-ounce) fresh cilantro

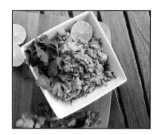

Procedure

1. Slice avocados in half, take the pitt out, and dice them inside the shell.
2. Slice red onion thin, dice jalapeno, and slice limes in half.
3. Combine all ingredients into a bowl and lightly mash avocado using a fork while mixing. Squeeze lime juice into   bowl.
4. Coarsely chop a half bunch of cilantro and add to the guacamole. Mix well until everything is combined.

Servings: makes 2 cups

https://www.ruled.me/instant-pot-artichoke-dip/

½ cup chicken broth

8 ounces cream cheese

10 ounce box frozen spinach

14 ounce can artichoke hearts, drained and chopped

½ cup sour cream

½ cup mayo

3 cloves garlic

1 teaspoon onion powder

12 ounces shredded Parmesan cheese

12 ounces shredded Swiss cheese

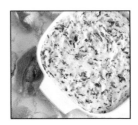

Procedure

Place all of the ingredients, except for the Parmesan and Swiss cheeses, into the Instant Pot.

Seal the lid and make sure that the vent is also sealed. Set it to pressure cooker, and set the timer for four minutes.

Once the timer is up, perform a manual release.

Add the cheeses into the instant pot and stir until everything is melted and gooey.

Serve right away with something for dipping, like pork rinds or kale chips.

Servings: 20

Low Carb Chocolate Chip Cookies

https://www.ruled.me/low-carb-chocolate-chip-cookies/

2½ cups almond flour
¼ cup walnuts, shelled and chopped
½ cup unsalted butter
2 large eggs
½ cup erythritol
½ cup dark chocolate chips
½ teaspoon salt
½ teaspoon baking soda
1 tablespoon vanilla extract

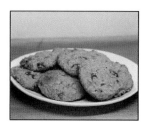

Procedure

Preheat oven to 350 F.

In a large bowl, combine almond flour, salt, baking soda, and erythritol.

In another bowl, melt butter and mix in vanilla, chocolate chips, eggs, and walnuts

Mix wet ingredients into the dry until a dough forms.

Scoop out 1 tbsp of dough per cookie and place onto a cookie sheet

Bake for 8-10 minutes, or until the edges have turned golden brown.

Remove from oven and transfer to a stable cooling rack to avoid crumbling. They firm as they cool.

Let cool for 10-15 minutes, then enjoy!

Servings: 18

https://www.ruled.me/keto-cream-cheese-truffles/

16 ounces cream cheese, softened
½ cup unsweetened cocoa powder, divided
4 tablespoons Swerve confectioners
¼ teaspoon liquid Stevia
½ teaspoon rum extract
1 tablespoon instant coffee
2 tablespoons water
1 tablespoon heavy whipping cream
24 paper candy cups for serving

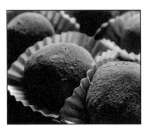

In a large bowl add the cream cheese, 1/4 cup of cocoa powder, Swerve, Stevia, rum extract, instant coffee, water, and heavy whipping cream.

Use an electric hand mixer to whip all of the ingredients together until they are well combined.

Place the bowl in the fridge for half an hour to chill before rolling.

Spread the remaining 1/4 cup cocoa powder out.

Roll heaping tablespoons in the palm of your hand to form balls, then roll them around in the cocoa powder. You will end up with about 24 total. Place them individually in small paper candy cups.

Chill for an hour before serving.

Servings: 24

Egg Salad Stuffed Avocados

https://www.ruled.me/egg-salad-stuffed-avocado/

6 large hard boiled eggs
⅓ medium red onion
3 ribs celery
4 tablespoons mayonnaise
2 teaspoons brown mustard
2 tablespoons fresh lime juice
1 teaspoon hot sauce
½ teaspoon cumin
Salt and pepper to taste
3 medium avocados

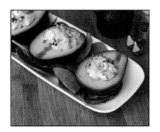

Procedure

1. Prep all ingredients by chopping eggs, onion, and celery.
2. Combine in a bowl with all of the ingredients except for avocado.
3. Slice avocado in half and take the pit out.
4. Spoon egg salad into avocado.

Servings: 6

https://www.ruled.me/oven-roasted-caprese-salad/

4 cloves garlic, peeled
3 cups grape tomatoes
2 tablespoons avocado oil
4 cups baby spinach leaves
10 pieces pearl size mozzarella balls
1 tablespoon pesto
1 tablespoon brine reserved from cheese
¼ cup fresh basil leaves

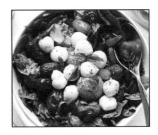

Procedure

Heat oven to 400°F and prepare a baking sheet with foil. Spread out the peeled garlic cloves and grape tomatoes evenly.

Drizzle avocado oil over the tomatoes and mix to coat.

Bake for 20-30 minutes or until the juices are released and the tops become slightly brown.

Drain the liquid from the mozzarella, reserving 1 tablespoon, and mix the tablespoon of brine with the pesto.

Remove the tomatoes from the oven and put the spinach in a large serving bowl.

Top the spinach with warm tomatoes and roasted garlic and drizzle with pesto sauce.

Add mozzarella balls and garnish with fresh torn basil leaves.

Servings: 4

https://www.ruled.me/cinnamon-roll-oatmeal/

1 cup crushed pecans
⅓ cup flax seed meal
⅓ cup chia seeds
½ cup riced cauliflower (~ 3 oz.)
3 ½ cups coconut milk
¼ cup heavy cream
3 ounces cream cheese
3 tablespoon butter
1 ½ teaspoons cinnamon
1 teaspoon maple flavor
½ teaspoon vanilla
¼ teaspoon nutmeg
¼ teaspoon allspice
3 tablespoons erythritol, powdered
10-15 drops liquid stevia
⅛ teaspoon xanthan gum

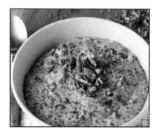

Rice cauliflower in a food processor and set aside.

Start heating coconut milk in a pan over medium heat.

Crush pecans and add to pan over low heat to toast.

Add cauliflower to coconut milk, bring to a boil, then reduce to simmer. Add spices and mix together.

Grind erythritol and add to the pan, then add the stevia, flax, and chia seeds. Mix this together as best you can.

Add cream, butter, and cream cheese to the pan and mix again. Add xanthan gum (optionally) if you want it a bit thicker.

Serving: 6

https://www.ruled.me/cinnamon-roll-pudding-pops/

As much or as little of this recipe as you want:

Cinnamon Roll 'Oatmeal'

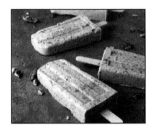

Procedure

Blend the Cinnamon Roll "Oatmeal" recipe in the blender.

Spoon mixture into the popsicle molds.

Insert spoon in and out of popsicle mold to get rid of any air bubbles, then put the lid on top.

Insert popsicle sticks and freeze for at least 3-4 hours.

Run a hot water bath in sink and submerge the molds into the hot water for 20-30 seconds.

Pull and wiggly popsicles to come out easily.

Servings: dependent on how much oatmeal you make
Each serving = ½ cup

https://www.ruled.me/raspberry-lemon-popsicles/

100g raspberries
½ lemon, juiced
¼ cup coconut oil
1 cup coconut milk
¼ cup sour cream
¼ cup heavy cream
½ teaspoon guar gum
20 drops liquid stevia

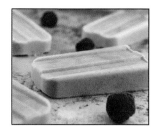

Procedure

1. Add all ingredients into a container and use an immersion blender (hand blender) to blend the mixture together.
2. Strain the mixture, discarding all raspberry seeds.
3. Pour the mixture into popsicle molds. Freeze for at least 2 hours.
4. Run the mold under hot water to dislodge the popsicles.

Servings: 6

https://www.ruled.me/peanut-butter-caramel-milkshake/

1 cup coconut milk (from the carton)
7 ice cubes
2 tablespoons peanut butter
2 tablespoons Torani Salted Caramel
1 tablespoon MCT oil
1/4 teaspoon xanthan gum

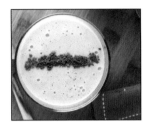

Procedure

Add all ingredients to your blender.
Blend everything together for 1-2 minutes or until the consistency is good for you
Pour out and enjoy! Add a little cocoa powder on top if you'd like..

Servings: 1

Blueberry Banana Bread Smoothie

https://www.ruled.me/blueberry-banana-bread-smoothie/

3 tablespoons golden flaxseed meal
1 tablespoon chia seeds
2 cups vanilla unsweetened coconut milk (from carton)
10 drops liquid stevia
¼ cup blueberries
2 tablespoons MCT oil
1 ½ teaspoons banana extract
¼ teaspoon xanthan gum

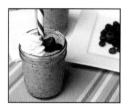

Procedure

Add all ingredients together into a blender. Wait a few minutes before blending, so that the flax and chia seeds have enough time to soak up some of the moisture.

Blend for 1-2 minutes until everything is incorporated well, then serve up!

Servings: 2

https://www.ruled.me/keto-mocha-ice-cream/

1 cup coconut milk (from the carton)
¼ cup heavy cream
2 tablespoons erythritol
15 drops liquid stevia
2 tablespoons cocoa powder
1 tablespoon instant coffee
¼ teaspoon xanthan gum

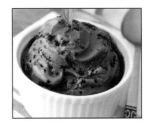

Add all ingredients except for xanthan gum into a container, then blend with an immersion blender (hand blender).

Slowly add in xanthan gum while blending until a slightly thicker mixture is formed.

Add to your ice cream machine and follow manufacturers instructions.

Servings: 2

https://www.ruled.me/keto-breakfast-tacos/

1 cup shredded mozzarella cheese
6 large eggs
2 tablespoons butter
3 strips bacon
½ small avocado
1 ounce cheddar cheese, shredded
Salt and pepper to taste

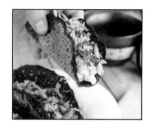

Procedure

1. Preheat oven to 375F.
2. Cook the bacon on a baking sheet with foil for about 15-20 minutes.
3. While the bacon is cooking, heat 1/3 cup of mozzarella at a time on clean pan on medium heat for the shells.
4. Wait until the cheese is browned on the edges (about 2-3 minutes).
5. Use a pair of tongs to lift the shell up and drape it over a wooden spoon resting on a pot. Do the same with the rest of your cheese, working in batches of 1/3 cups.
6. Cook your eggs in the butter, stirring occasionally until they're done. Season with salt and pepper.
7. Spoon a third of your scrambled eggs, avocado, and bacon into each hardened taco shell.
8. Sprinkle cheddar cheese over the tops of the breakfast tacos. Add hot sauce and cilantro if you'd like!

Servings: 3

https://www.drberg.com/Ketogenic-diet-meals-recipes/breakfast/keto-friendly-fluffy-pancakes

1 cup almond flour
1 tablespoon xylitol (powdered)
½ teaspoon baking powder
¼ teaspoon baking soda
1 pinch, sea salt, finely ground
½ cup buttermilk
1 large egg
1 tablespoon light olive oil
Serve with softened butter or maple syrup

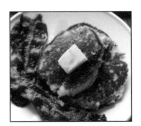

Procedure

Mix together dry ingredients: almond flour, xylitol, baking powder, baking soda, and salt.

In a separate bowl, mix together wet ingredients: buttermilk, egg, light olive oil.

Gently mix wet ingredients into the dry ingredients.

Set pan or griddle to medium heat (350 degrees). Make into 6 medium pancakes. Smaller pancakes are easier to flip.

Servings: 6

https://www.drberg.com/Ketogenic-diet-meals-recipes/breakfast/keto-waffles

1 cup almond flour
1 pinch salt
1 teaspoon baking soda
4 eggs
¼ cup Fiber Yum
Cooking spray (Avocado spray works great!)

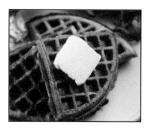

Procedure

Heat waffle iron per the directions that came with it. Spray both sides of iron with oil before batter is poured in.

Mix all ingredients above. Do not over mix.

Pour batter in and cook per the directions that came with your waffle iron. All are different!

Best served right away. If not, put on a cookie sheet, and don't stack. They tend to get soft when stacked.

Add butter and sugar free syrup or peanut butter and enjoy!

Servings: 4 waffle halves

https://www.drberg.com/Ketogenic-diet-meals-recipes/lunch_dinner/tuna-cakes

¼ cup almond flour

2.5 ounces tuna

1 large egg

2 cups cabbage

3 each scallions

2 tablespoons mayonnaise

2 tablespoons apple cider vinegar

1 teaspoon salt

1 tablespoon olive oil

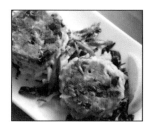

Cut up cabbage. Mix together mayo, cabbage, apple cider vinegar, 1 scallion, and salt. Place cabbage in refrigerator for at least 30 minutes.

Mix together almond flour, egg, tuna, and 2 scallions in a bowl. Divide into 3 equal parts. Form into patties.

Put oil in pan, turn on medium high heat.

Gently place tuna patties into hot oil. Let cook on one side without touching for 3 minutes on medium heat.

This will form a crispy delicious sear. Flip and cook the other side for 3 more minutes.

Place patties on paper towel on a plate to absorb the oil.

Serve on top of coleslaw!

Servings: 1

https://www.drberg.com/Ketogenic-diet-meals-recipes/lunch_dinner/tuna-cabbage-casserole

2.5 ounce can tuna, drained
1 ½ cups cabbage
1 cup cauliflower
1 tablespoon olive oil
1 tablespoon butter
1 tablespoon heavy whipping cream
1 ounce mozzarella

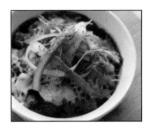

Procedure

1. Preheat oven to 350F.
2. Chop cabbage and cauliflower.
3. Add oil to pan, turn to medium high heat. Once pan is hot, add cauliflower and cabbage. Saute on medium high for 5-7 minutes until cauliflower gets a little golden.
4. Add tuna, butter, cream. Cook on low for 2-3 mins.
5. Put mixture into a small casserole dish.
6. Cover casserole dish with mozzarella cheese.
7. Bake in oven for 15-20 mins.
8. Garnish with parmesan cheese for extra cheesiness and some shaved vegetables for extra crunch!

Servings: 1

https://www.drberg.com/Ketogenic-diet-meals-recipes/lunch_dinner/pepperoni-cheese-fat-bomb

3.5 ounce cream cheese, ½ cup at room temp
2 ounce butter, ¼ cup at room temperature
¼ cup pepperoni (2 oz)
2 tablespoon cheddar cheese (1 oz), shredded
2 cloves garlic
1 cup parmesan cheese, grated
2-3 leaves basil

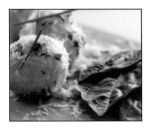

Dice pepperoni. Cook at medium-low heat for 5-8 minutes. Remove from heat. Place on paper towel to soak up extra grease.

Mix together cream cheese, butter, cheddar cheese.

Add garlic. Fold in pepperoni.

Divide mixture into 6 equal parts.

Grate parmesan and chop basil, place into a separate bowl.

Place one fat bomb at a time in the bowl to coat it in the parmesan and basil.

Servings: 6

https://recipes.mercola.com/chicken-oregano-recipe.aspx

4-5 chicken breasts from organic, free-range chickens
1 large head fresh cauliflower, sectioned into florets
2 lemons (½ cup juice)
½ cup coconut oil
1 cup organic bone broth or chicken stock
3 tablespoons organic dried oregano
1 pinch of paprika, optional
2 teaspoons himalayan salt

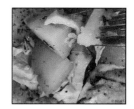

Procedure

Preheat oven to 350F.

In a roasting pot with lid, add chicken and cauliflower and season well with himalayan salt, pepper and paprika.

In a separate bowl, combine lemon juice, coconut oil, bone broth, oregano, sea salt and whisk together briskly.

Pour liquid mixture over chicken (it should cover the chicken; you can add more broth if needed).

Cover and cook for 45 minutes.

Servings: 4

https://recipes.mercola.com/crock-pot-chicken-noodle-soup-recipe.aspx

2 organic, pasture raised chicken breasts
2 tablespoons coconut oil
3 full size organic carrots, sliced
2 organic celery stalks, sliced
1 organic yellow onion, diced
2 tablespoons fresh parsley
2 organic zucchini
½ teaspoon dried thyme
64 ounces chicken broth
Salt and pepper to taste

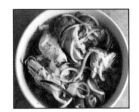

Procedure

Cut ends of zucchini; place zucchini through the spiralizer to create zucchini noodles.

Drizzle crockpot with coconut oil.

Place chicken at the bottom of the pot, and then top with carrots, celery, zucchini noodles, thyme, chicken broth, salt and pepper.

Cook on high for 4 hours.

Chicken should now be easy to cut. Serve the noodle soup in bowls. Add more salt and pepper to taste.

Servings: 3-4

INDEX

Alcohol / Spirits (Gin, Rum, Vodka, Whiskey)	28,31
Alfalfa Sprouts, raw	11,31
Almond Butter, unsalted	16,31
Almond Milk, plain, unsweetened	14,31
Almonds, nuts, raw, unsalted, single	20,31
American Cheese, single slice	15,31
Anchovies, canned, pieces	17,31
Apple Juice or Cider, unsweetened	20,31
Apple, raw, w/o skin, single	20,31
Apple, raw, w/skin, single	20,31
Apricots, dried	20,31
Apricots, raw, single	20,31
Artichokes, fresh, boiled, single	11,31
Artichokes, raw, single	11,31
Arugula, raw	11,31
Asparagus, fresh or frozen, boiled	11,31
Asparagus, raw, single spear	11,31
Avocado, black, single	20,31
Bacon, single slice	19,31
Bacon and Roasted Garlic Guacamole (Recipe)	52
Bagel, plain, single	22,31
Baking powder	24,31
Baking soda	24,31
Bamboo shoots, raw	11,31
Banana, raw, single	21,31
Barley, pearled, cooked	22,31
Basil, dried	26,31
Bass, 3 oz fillet	17,31
BBQ sauce, homemade	23,31
Bean sprouts, mung, raw	11,31
Beer, light	27,32
Beer, reg	27,32

Beets, fresh, boiled	11,32
Beets, raw, single	11,32
Biscuit, homemade, single	22,32
Bison, steak, 3 oz	17,32
Black Beans, canned, drained	19,32
Black Beans, dry, cooked	19,32
Black Pepper, ground	24,32
Blackberries, frozen	21,32
Blackberries, raw, single	21,32
Blue Cheese Dressing	16,32
Blue Cheese, crumbled	15,32
Blueberries, frozen	21,32
Blueberries, raw, single	21,32
Blueberry Banana Bread Smoothie (Recipe)	63
Bok Choy, shredded	11,32
Bologna, single slice	19,32
Bone Broth, beef	28,32
Bone Broth, chicken	28,32
Bratwurst, sausage, single link	19,32
Brazil Nuts, raw, unsalted, single	20,32
Bread crumbs, plain	24,32
Bread, wheat, single slice	22,32
Bread, white, gluten free, single slice	22,32
Bread, white, single slice	22,32
Bread, zero carb, single slice	22,32
Breakfast bars, most, single	27,32
Brick Cheese, single cracker slice	15,32
Brie Cheese	15,32
Broccoli, fresh, boiled, chopped	11,33
Broccoli, raw, chopped	11,33
Broccoli, raw, single flower	11,33
Brownie, chocolate, single	27,33
Brussel Sprouts, fresh, boiled, whole	11,33

Brussel Sprouts, raw, pieces	11,33
Butter, cashew, unsalted	16,33
Butter, ghee	16,33
Butter, margarine	16,33
Butter, peanut, organic, no stir	16,33
Butter, raw, salted	16,33
Butter, sunflower seed	16,33
Butter, tahini, sesame seed butter	16,33
Buttermilk, whole	14,33
Cabbage, green, fresh, cooked	11,33
Cabbage, green, raw, chopped	11,33
Cabbage, red, fresh, cooked	11,33
Cabbage, red, raw, chopped	11,33
Cacoa powder	24,33
Caesar Dressing	16,33
Cake, piece or cupcake, single	27,33
Calamari, squid, breaded	17,33
Canola Oil	16,33
Cantaloupe, melon, cubed	21,33
Carrots, baby, raw, single	11,33
Carrots, fresh, cooked, diced	11,33
Carrots, fresh, single	11,33
Cashew Milk, plain, unsweetened	14,33
Cashews, nuts, raw, unsalted, single	20,33
Catfish, 6 oz fillet	18,33
Cauliflower, fresh, boiled	11,34
Cauliflower, raw, single flower	11,34
Caviar	18,34
Cayenne Pepper	26,34
Celery, fresh, cooked	11,34
Celery, raw, single stalk	11,34
Cheddar Cheese, shredded	15,34
Cheddar Cheese, single cracker slice	15,34

Index	Page
Cheesecake, single slice	27,34
Cherries, frozen	21,34
Cherries, sweet, pitted, single	21,34
Chia Seeds	20,34
Chicken, breast, baked or roasted, 1/2 breast	17,34
Chicken, canned, 5 oz	19,34
Chicken, cornish game hen, roasted, 3 oz	17,34
Chicken, leg, breaded and fried	17,34
Chicken, whole, roasted, 3 oz	17,34
Chicken Oregano (Recipe)	71
Chili Powder	26,34
Chocolate Chip Cookies, single	27,34
Chocolate Milk, whole	14,34
Cilantro, raw, single sprig	11,34
Cinnamon	26,34
Cinnamon Roll 'Oatmeal' (Recipe)	59
Cinnamon Roll Pudding Pops (Recipe)	60
Clams, fresh, cooked, single	18,34
Clementine, single	21,34
Cloves, ground	26,34
Cocoa powder	24,34
Coconut Milk, canned, unsweetened	21,34
Coconut Oil	16,34
Coconut Water	21,34
Coconut, whole, single	21,34
Cod, 4 oz fillet	18,35
Coffee Cream, powdered	14,35
Coffee, ground, decaf	27,35
Coffee, ground, reg	27,35
Colby Cheese, single slice	15,35
Coleslaw	23,35
Collagen Powder	28,35
Collards, fresh, cooked	12,35

Condensed milk, sweetened	24,35
Cooking spray	24,35
Corn Oil	16,35
Corn starch	25,35
Corn syrup	25,35
Corn, canned, cream	12,35
Corn, canned, whole	12,35
Corn, frozen, whole kernel	12,35
Corn, single ear, cooked	12,35
Corn, single ear, raw	12,35
Corned Beef, single slice	19,35
Cornmeal	25,35
Cottage Cheese, 2%	15,35
Cottage Cheese, whole	15,35
Crab leg, single	18,35
Crab meat	18,35
Cranberries, dried, sweetened	21,35
Cranberry Juice, unsweetened	21,35
Crayfish or crawfish	18,35
Cream Cheese	15,35
Crockpot Chicken Noodle Soup (Recipe)	72
Croissant Roll, single	23,35
Croutons, seasoned, 1 svg of 7g	23,35
Cucumber, raw, single slice	12,36
Cumin	26,36
Dates, pitted, medjool, single	21,36
Deli Meat, turkey, single slice	19,36
Dinner Roll, sweet, single	23,36
Dinner Roll, wheat, single	23,36
Donut, cake, chocolate frosted, single	27,36
Donut, glazed, single	27,36
Doritos, chips, single	26,36
Edam Cheese, single cracker slice	15,36

Edamame, fresh, cooked	12,36
Egg, substitute, white, single	14,36
Egg, white, cooked, single	14,36
Egg, whole, raw or cooked, single	14,36
Egg, yolk, cooked, single	14,36
Egg Salad Stuffed Avocados (Recipe)	57
Eggplant, fresh, cooked	12,36
Eggplant, raw, peeled, single	12,36
English Muffin, wheat, single whole	23,36
English Muffin, white, single whole	23,36
Erythritol	25,36
Evaporated milk	25,36
Fennel, raw, sliced	12,36
Feta Cheese, crumbled	15,36
Figs, dried, single	21,36
Figs, raw, single	21,36
Fish sticks, single stick	18,36
Flank, steak, 3 oz	17,36
Flaxseed Oil	16,36
Flaxseed, ground	25,36
Flaxseeds, raw	20,36
Flour, all purpose white	25,37
Flour, almond	25,37
Flour, coconut	25,37
Flour, wheat	25,37
French Fries, potatoes, baked, steak, single	13,37
French Fries, potatoes, fried, single	13,37
French Toast, white, homemade, single	23,37
Garbanzo Beans (chick peas), canned, drained	19,37
Garbanzo Beans (chick peas), dry, cooked	19,37
Garlic Powder	26,37
Garlic, minced	26,37
Garlic, raw, single clove	12,37

Index	Page
Gin	28,37
Goat Cheese, soft, crumbled	15,37
Goat Milk	14,37
Gouda Cheese, single cracker slice	15,37
Grape, juice, unsweetened	21,37
Grapefruit, juice	21,37
Grapefruit, raw, single	21,37
Grapes, raw, seedless, single	21,37
Green Beans, snap, fresh, cooked	11,37
Green Beans, snap, raw, single	11,37
Green Onions, (scallions), tops and bulb, raw, single	12,37
Ground beef, 85% lean	17,37
Gruyere Cheese, single cracker slice	15,37
Guacamole	23,37
Haddock, 7 oz fillet	18,37
Half and Half, cream	14,37
Halibut, 26 oz	18,37
Ham, honey roasted, 2 oz	19,37
Hamburger/Hot Dog Bun, wheat, single	23,38
Hamburger/Hot Dog Bun, white, single	23,38
Hashbrowns, potatoes	13,38
Hazelnuts, nuts, single	20,38
Herring, 7 oz fillet	18,38
Honey, raw	25,38
Horseradish	23,38
Hot Chocolate or Hot Cocoa	27,38
Hot Pepper Sauce	23,38
Hummus	23,38
Ice Cream, most flavors	27,38
Instant Pot Artichoke Dip (Recipe)	54
Italian Dressing	16,38
Italian Sausage, single link	19,38
Jalapeno Peppers, canned	13,38

Index	Page
Jalapeno Peppers, raw, single	13,38
Jello, flavored, sugar free, single container	27,38
Jelly, grape, squeezable	16,38
Jicama, cooked	12,38
Jicama, raw, sliced	12,38
Kale, fresh, cooked	12,38
Kale, raw	12,38
Kefir, lowfat, flavored	15,38
Kefir, whole, plain	15,38
Ketchup (Catsup)	24,38
Keto Breakfast Tacos (Recipe)	65
Keto Cream Cheese Truffles (Recipe)	56
Keto Friendly Fluffy Pancakes (Recipe)	66
Keto Mocha Ice Cream (Recipe)	64
Keto Waffles (Recipe)	67
Kidney Beans, canned, drained	19,38
Kidney Beans, dry, cooked	19,38
Kiwi, raw, single	21,38
Kombucha Tea, cranberry flavored	27,38
Lard (made from animal fats)	16,38
Leeks, fresh, cooked, single	12,39
Leeks, raw, single	12,39
Lemon, juice	21,39
Lemon, raw, single	21,39
Lentil Beans, canned, drained	19,39
Lentil Beans, dry, cooked	19,39
Lettuce, Boston, Bib, Butterhead	12,39
Lettuce, Iceberg	12,39
Lettuce, Romaine	12,39
Lime, raw, single	21,39
Liverwurst, sausage, single slice	19,39
Lobster, 1 lb	18,39
Low Carb Chocolate Chip Cookies	55

Macadamia Nuts, single	20,39
Mackerel, 8 oz fillet	18,39
Mango, raw, single	21,39
Mashed Potatoes	13,39
Mayonnaise	24,39
MCT Oil	28,39
MCT Oil, powder	28,39
Melba Toast, single	26,39
Melon, honeydew, cubed	21,39
Milk, cow, 2%	14,39
Milk, cow, whole	14,39
Miso	24,39
Mixed nuts, dry, roasted, salted, single	20,39
Molasses, dark or light	25,39
Mozzarella Cheese, part skim, shredded	15,39
Muffin, bran, single	27,39
Mushrooms, canned	12,39
Mushrooms, fresh, cooked	12,39
Mushrooms, raw, single	12,40
Mustard Greens, fresh, cooked	12,40
Mustard, dried	26,40
Mustard, sauce	24,40
Navy Beans, canned, drained	19,40
Navy Beans, dry, cooked	19,40
Nectarine, raw, single	21,40
Nutella	16,40
Nutmeg	26,40
Oatmeal Cookies, single	27,40
Oatmeal, cooked	23,40
Okra, fresh, cooked	12,40
Olive Oil, extra virgin, cold pressed	16,40
Olives, black, raw, single	12,40
Olives, green, raw, single	12,40

Onion Dip	24,40
Onion Powder	26,40
Onions, green (scallions), tops & bulb, single	12,40
Onions, white, yellow, red, fresh, cooked	12,40
Onions, white, yellow, red, raw, single	13,40
Orange Juice	22,40
Orange, raw, single	22,40
Oregano, dried	26,40
Oven Roasted Caprese Salad (Recipe)	58
Oreos, cookies, single	27,40
Oysters, canned, 8 oz	18,40
Oysters, fresh, cooked	18,40
Paleo Egg Bake (Recipe)	51
Pan Tuna Cakes (Recipe)	68
Pancake, homemade, single	23,40
Papaya, raw, single	22,40
Parmesan Cheese, fresh or dry, grated	15,40
Parsley, dried	26,40
Parsley, raw	13,40
Parsnip, cooked, single	13,41
Pasta Noodles, cooked	23,41
Pastrami, beef, single slice	19,41
Pea Protein, powder	28,41
Peach, raw, single	22,41
Peanut Butter Caramel Milkshake (Recipe)	62
Peanut Oil	16,41
Peanuts, nuts, single	20,41
Pear, raw, single	22,41
Peas, green, canned	13,41
Peas, green, fresh or frozen, cooked	13,41
Peas, snowpeas, raw, single pod	13,41
Pecans, nuts, single	20,41
Pepperoni Cheese Fat Bomb (Recipe)	70
Perch, 2 oz fillet	18,41

Pesto, homemade	24,41
Pickle, single slice	24,41
Pickle, sour, single whole	24,41
Pie, chocolate cream, single crust, single slice	27,41
Pie, fruit, double crust, single slice	27,41
Pike, 26 oz fillet	18,41
Pine Nuts	20,41
Pineapple Juice	22,41
Pineapple, raw, chunks	22,41
Pinto Beans, canned, drained	20,41
Pinto Beans, dry, cooked	20,41
Pistachios, nuts, single	20,41
Pita, white, single	23,41
Pita, whole grain, single	23,41
Plantain, raw, single	22,41
Plum, raw, single	22,41
Polish Kielbasa, sausage, single link	19,41
Pomegranate, raw, single	22,42
Popcorn, home, air popped	26,42
Popcorn, microwave	26,42
Pork, chops, single	17,42
Pork, ground	17,42
Pork, loin, 3 oz	17,42
Pork, ribs, spare, single	17,42
Potato Chips, single	26,42
Potato Salad, homemade	24,42
Potato, baked, skin not eaten, single	13,42
Potato, boiled w/o skin, single	13,42
Prune Juice, unsweetened	22,42
Prunes, dried	22,42
Psyllium Husk Powder	25,42
Pudding, chocolate	27,42
Pudding, chocolate, sugar free	27,42
Pumpkin Seeds, raw, unsalted	20,42

Quinoa, cooked	23,42
Radish, raw, single	13,42
Raisins, uncooked	22,42
Ranch Dressing, creamy	16,42
Raspberries, raw, single	22,42
Raspberry Lemon Popsicles (Recipe)	61
Relish, sweet pickle	24,42
Rhubarb, cooked, unsweetened	22,42
Rhubarb, raw, stalk	22,42
Rib roast, 3 oz	17,42
Ribeye, 4 oz	17,42
Rice Milk, plain, unsweetened	14,42
Rice, brown, cooked	23,42
Rice, white, cooked	23,42
Ricotta Cheese, part skim	15,43
Ricotta Cheese, whole	15,43
Ritz Crackers, single	26,43
Romano Cheese, fresh or dry, grated	15,43
Rosemary, dried	26,43
Round roast, 3 oz	17,43
Rum	28,43
Rump roast, 4 oz	17,43
Safflower Oil	16,43
Salami, pork and beef, single slice	19,43
Salmon, wild alaskan, canned	18,43
Salmon, wild alaskan, fresh	18,43
Salsa	24,43
Salt, garlic	26,43
Salt, iodized	26,43
Salt, onion	26,43
Salt, sea	26,43
Saltines, crackers, single	26,43
Sardines, canned, water, 4 oz	18,43
Sauerkraut	24,43

Sausage, breakfast, single patty	19,43
Scallops	18,43
Seaweed, dulse, dried	13,43
Sesame Oil	16,43
Sherbet	27,43
Short ribs, 3 oz	17,43
Shrimp, breaded	18,43
Shrimp, frozen	18,43
Simple, Delicious Guacamole (Recipe)	53
Sirloin, 3 oz	17,43
Smelt	18,43
Snapper, 8 oz fillet	18,44
Soda, club	28,44
Soda, dark, diet	28,44
Soda, dark, reg	28,44
Soda, light, diet	28,44
Soda, light, reg	28,44
Sour Cream	14,44
Soy Milk, plain, unsweetened	14,44
Soy Sauce	24,44
Spaghetti Sauce, homemade	24,44
Spinach, canned	13,44
Spinach, frozen, cooked	13,44
Spinach, raw	13,44
Spirulina, seaweed, raw	13,44
Sports drink (gatorade)	28,44
Squash, butternut, baked	13,44
Squash, spaghetti, baked	13,44
Stevia, drops	25,44
Stevia, packets, single	25,44
Stew beef, cubed	17,44
Strawberries, frozen, unsweetened	22,44
Strawberries, raw, single	22,44

Sugar, brown, packed	25,44
Sugar, white, granulated, cooking	25,44
Sugar, white, granulated, sweetening	25,44
Sugar, white, powdered	25,44
Summer Sausage, beef, single slice	19,44
Sunflower Oil	16,44
Sunflower Seeds	20,44
Sweet Peppers, fresh, cooked, chopped	13,45
Sweet Peppers, raw, single	13,45
Sweet Potato (yam), baked, single	13,45
Swiss Cheese, single slice	15,45
Syrup, maple, organic	24,45
Syrup, pancake	24,45
T-bone, 4 oz	17,45
Tangerine (mandarin), raw, single	22,45
Tartar Sauce	24,45
Tea, brewed, unsweetened	28,45
Tea, iced, lemon, unsweetened	28,45
Tempeh, single patty	20,45
Tenderloin, 3 oz	17,45
Thyme, dried	26,45
Tofu, single slice	20,45
Tomato Sauce	24,45
Tomato, canned	13,45
Tomato, cherry, single	13,45
Tomato, fresh, cooked	13,45
Tomato, raw, single	13,45
Tomato, sundried, jar w/oil	13,45
Tortilla Chips, single	26,45
Tortilla, corn, single	23,45
Tortilla, flour, single	23,45
Trout, rainbow, 3 oz fillet	18,45
Tuna, steaks, 5 oz	18,45

Tuna, white, canned, 5 oz	18,45
Tuna Cabbage Casserole (Recipe)	69
Turkey, ground	17,45
Turkey, whole, roasted, 3 oz	17,45
Turnip, fresh, cooked, single	14,46
Turnip, raw, single	14,46
Vanilla extract	25,46
Vanilla Wafer, cookies, single	27,46
Veal, cutlets, 3 oz	17,46
Veal, ground	17,46
Vegetable Juice Cocktail	28,46
Vegetable Oil	16,46
Venison, stew meat	17,46
Vienna Sausage, single link	19,46
Vinaigrette Dressing, oil	16,46
Vinegar, apple cider	25,46
Vinegar, rice wine	25,46
Vinegar, white distilled	25,46
Vodka	28,46
Waffle, homemade, single	23,46
Waffle, plain, frozen, single	23,46
Walleye, 6 oz fillet	18,46
Walnut Oil	16,46
Walnuts, nuts, single halves	20,46
Water, Zero, flavored	28,46
Watercress, raw	14,46
Watermelon, cubed	21,46
Weiner, hot dog, single link	19,46
Whey Protein powder	28,46
Whipping Cream, heavy	14,46
Whiskey	28,46
White Beans, canned, drained	20,46
White Beans, dry, cooked	20,46

Whitefish, 7 oz fillet	18,46
Wine, dessert, sweet	28,47
Wine, table, red	28,47
Wine, table, white	28,47
Worcheshire Sauce	24,47
Xylitol	25,47
Yeast, baking, active dry	25,47
Yogurt, greek, nonfat, plain	15,47
Yogurt, lowfat, flavored	15,47
Yogurt, lowfat, plain	15,47
Yogurt, plain, whole	15,47
Zucchini, fresh, cooked	14,47
Zucchini, raw, single	14,47

38342460R00056

Printed in Poland
by Amazon Fulfillment
Poland Sp. z o.o., Wrocław